SECOND EDITION

EXERCISES IN DIAGNOSTIC RADIOLOGY

5

PEDIATRICS

RICHARD M. HELLER, M.D.

Professor of Radiology and Radiological Sciences
Head, Section of Pediatric Radiology
Professor of Pediatrics
Vanderbilt University Hospital
Nashville, Tennessee

SANDRA G. KIRCHNER, M.D.

Professor of Radiology
Associate Professor of Pediatrics
Section of Pediatric Radiology
Vanderbilt University Hospital
Nashville, Tennessee

GADI HOREV, M.D.

Fellow in Pediatric Radiology
Section of Pediatric Radiology and Radiological Sciences
Vanderbilt University Hospital
Nashville, Tennessee

LUCY FRANK SQUIRE, M.D.

Professor of Radiology
Downstate Medical Center
Brooklyn, New York
Consultant in Radiology
Massachusetts General Hospital
Boston, Massachusetts

D1522983

W. B. SAUNDERS COMPANY • 1987
Harcourt Brace Jovanovich, Inc.

Philadelphia • London • Toronto • Montreal • Sydney • Tokyo

W. B. Saunders Company: West Washington Square
                          Philadelphia, PA   19105

Library of Congress Cataloging-in-Publication Data
(Rev. for vol. 5)

Exercises in diagnostic radiology.

Includes indexes.

Contents: v. 1. The chest—[etc.]— v. 5. Pediatrics—v. 6.
  Nuclear imaging. 1. Diagnosis, Radioscopic—Programmed
  instruction. I. Squire, Lucy Frank.

RC78.E893 1981   616.07'57   81–51075

ISBN 0–7216–8543–O (pbk. : set)

Editor: William Lamsback
Designer: Karen O'Keefe
Production Manager: Bob Butler
Manuscript Editor: Tom Stringer
Illustration Coordinator: Walt Verbitski
Indexer: Susan Thomas

Listed here is the latest translated edition of this book together
with the language of the translation and the publisher.

French (Vol. V) (*1st Edition*)—Librairie Maloine, Paris, France
German (*1st Edition*)—Georg Thieme Verlag, Stuttgart, Germany
Spanish (*1st Edition*)—Nueva Editorial Interamericana, S.A. de C.V.
Japanese (*1st Edition*)—Hirokawa Publishing Co., Tokyo, Japan
Italian (*1st Edition*)—Piccin Editore, Padova, Italy

Exercises in Diagnostic Radiology—Volume 5 Pediatrics   ISBN 0–7216–1569–4

Last digit is the print number: 9   8   7   6   5   4   3   2   1

PREFACE

The task of preparing a second edition to *Exercises in Diagnostic Radiology, Pediatrics* has proved to be a challenging endeavor. We have had the opportunity to review the first edition, to judge which concepts have withstood the test of time and which concepts needed revision or deletion, and finally to introduce the use of new imaging methodologies. In the anticipation of this second edition, the team of authors reviewed publications on pediatric radiology that have appeared since the first edition and are convinced that *Exercises in Diagnostic Radiology* remains a useful tool for the education of medical students and house officers in the discipline of pediatric radiology. It is no accident that the case history format and quiz have been retained. Although illustrations have been replaced and text has been added to improve the second edition, our focus hasn't changed.

As pediatric radiology is an evolving discipline that includes not only conventional radiology but also magnetic resonance imaging, x-ray computed tomography, and ultrasound, where appropriate we have introduced these newer imaging methodologies. However, the importance of conventional imaging and a sound knowledge of clinical pediatrics in the practice of diagnostic pediatric radiology is stressed. As we look at the completed manuscript, we hope that we have provided an educational experience for the student of our discipline.

RICHARD M. HELLER
SANDRA G. KIRCHNER
GADI HOREV
LUCY FRANK SQUIRE

ACKNOWLEDGMENTS

The authors would like to take the opportunity to express their gratitude for support from their pediatric colleagues at the Children's Hospital of Vanderbilt University Medical Center, Chairman, Dr. David Karzon. In addition, we are grateful to Dr. Wallace (Skip) Neblett, Chairman of Pediatric Surgery, and to many pediatricians in private practice in middle Tennessee who have also allowed us to publish radiographs on their patients.

We are thankful for the support of Dr. A. Everette James, Jr., the Chairman of the Department of Radiology and Radiological Sciences at Vanderbilt University Medical Center. Archival assistance was provided by Nancy Hanna and Jim Brice; the photographs were made by John Bobbitt; and the manuscript was typed by Annette Allen and Lavonne Harris.

PREFACE TO THE FIRST EDITION

Children are not just small adults. They do have some of the diseases of adults, to be sure, although even these tend to be altered by the growth and metabolism peculiar to childhood. In addition there is a spectrum of disease conditions limited to the pediatric age group with its own radiologic patterns, evolving in our understanding as the subspecialty, pediatric radiology. It is as complex and as fascinating as the general field of radiology or any of its other subspecialties.

Several decades ago, the superb textbook of Dr. John Caffey appeared (*Pediatric X-Ray Diagnosis*, published by Year Book), and has ever since lead the field as an encyclopedic teaching and reference work. The authors' intention in producing this little volume is to present in problem format some of the highlights of the pediatric radiologic discipline. The problems and answers are offered to medical students, pediatric house officers, and radiology residents with the conviction that the subjects chosen are suitable for inclusion in board examinations and are common enough to be recognized at the end of training in either pediatrics or general radiology.

A conscious attempt has been made not to duplicate material already presented in the earlier volumes of this series, particularly in the section on Bone Growth in Volume 3. As indicated in the table of contents, the book is subdivided into groups of problems relating to the pediatric chest, abdomen, brain, and bones. Names and some details of the presenting histories have been altered, but the clinical facts of the cases are true.

As with the other volumes, we will be grateful for ideas and suggestions from our readers.

RICHARD M. HELLER

CONTENTS

Chest

FOUR PATIENTS WITH DIETARY INDISCRETION

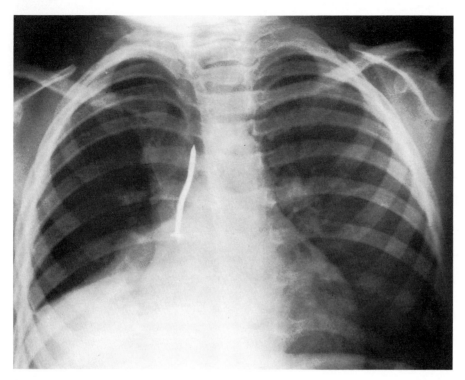

Figure 1. Rusty N.

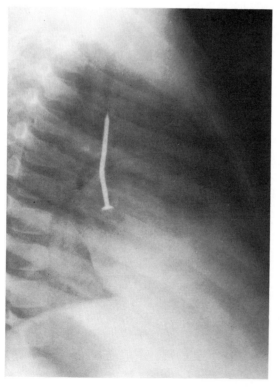

Figure 2. Rusty N.

Rusty N., a 3 year old girl, is brought by her mother to the Emergency Room because of a cough of three weeks' duration. This cough is worse at night, keeping the mother awake. Her mother wants *Rusty* to have a shot of penicillin and some cough medicine.

Physical examination shows reduced breath sounds in the distribution of the right lower lobe and right middle lobe. No rales are heard, but rhonchi are present. Her temperature is normal. You send *Rusty* to the Radiology Department for PA and lateral chest radiographs.

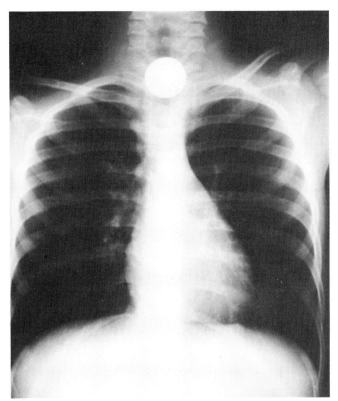

Figure 3. Argentia

Argentia, a 6 year old girl who stored objects in her mouth like a squirrel, laughed, choked, and her treasure disappeared. Where will you find it?

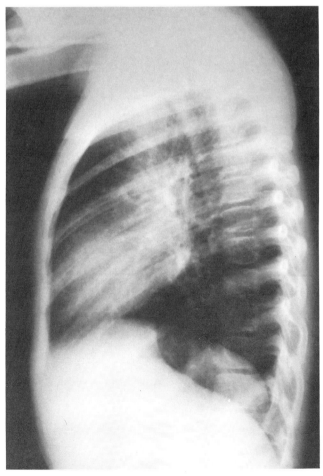

Figure 4. Argentia

ANSWERS

Rusty's chest radiographs show a nail directed vertically and toward the right. Its position so far off the midline indicates that it's not in the esophagus, but instead is in the trachea and right main stem bronchus. The lateral view is not straight, and you can see that one bronchus is normal and the other needs rust inhibitor. The lateral view also shows increased radiodensity in the right middle lobe area, and you can only see one hemidiaphragm. This indicates that the nail must be occluding the bronchus intermedius to the right middle and right lower lobes, resulting in atelectasis of these lobes. The right upper lobe bronchus must be patent; otherwise, there would be complete atelectasis of the right lung.

Bronchoscopy was performed, and the nail was removed. Unfortunately, over the next several months *Rusty* had recurrent pneumonias in the areas that had been atelectatic. The child stopped gaining weight and growing. During one of her asymptomatic periods, it was elected to perform a bronchogram (Fig. 5).

This study shows cylindrical dilation of the right lower and middle lobe bronchi. In the right upper lobe bronchus the normal tapering of the bronchi is seen as they progress toward the periphery of the lung.

The dilation of the bronchi, or bronchiectasis, is the result of obstruction of the bronchi, stasis of secretions, and infection that destroys the bronchial walls.

If the changes in the bronchi are mild and the obstruction is relieved promptly, the bronchiectasis may be reversible. *Rusty's* bronchiectasis was too advanced, and a right middle and right lower lobectomy had to be performed.

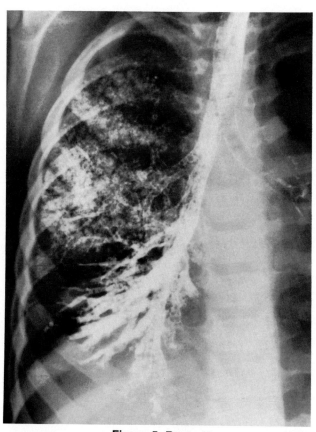

Figure 5. Rusty N.

She has done well since surgery and has exhibited normal growth and development.

Since *Argentia's* treasure didn't pop out of her mouth, it must have passed into either the trachea or the esophagus, and a chest radiograph would be the first study to request. Of course, you would ask for a frontal view, but is a lateral view also necessary? Actually no, if, as is suspected, the treasure is a coin! Recall that the esophagus is elliptical in the coronal plane, while the trachea is elliptical in the sagittal plane. This anatomy then explains the fact that coins in the trachea orient themselves with their long dimension anteroposterior, and coins in the esophagus orient themselves with their long dimension right to left. So in this case, *Argentia's* treasure is in the esophagus because it is seen "en face" on the frontal chest radiograph.

Now the question is how to retrieve *Argentia's* coin. In the past, endoscopy under general anesthesia was performed to remove esophageal foreign bodies. Today, in many institutions a radiologist can remove an esophageal coin by placing a Foley catheter beyond it and inflating the balloon under fluoroscopic control. With the child in the prone, oblique position, the coin is pulled into the mouth by withdrawal of the inflated balloon. It is important that the fluoroscopic table be tilted steeply so that the patient's head is lower than the body. This prevents aspiration of the coin into the airway. This extraction procedure is performed on outpatients and does not require anesthesia; however, it shouldn't be done if the foreign body has been lodged in the esophagus for longer than 24 to 48 hours because of the risk of mediastinitis.

Argentia's major concern was the return of the coin. Would you give it back to her? We did that once, and never will again—we had to retrieve the coin a second time!

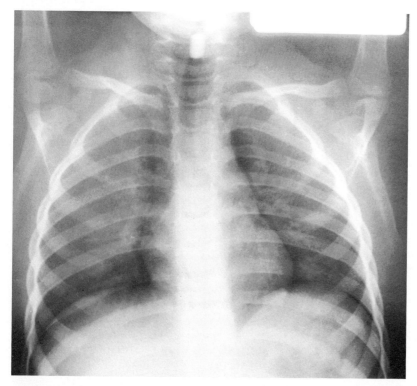

Figure 6. Demosthenes

Here is our friend **Demosthenes,** who is a budding, 3 year old orator. Unfortunately, one less object was removed from his mouth than he inserted. Where did it go? Illustrated here are two frontal chest radiographs taken within minutes of each other.

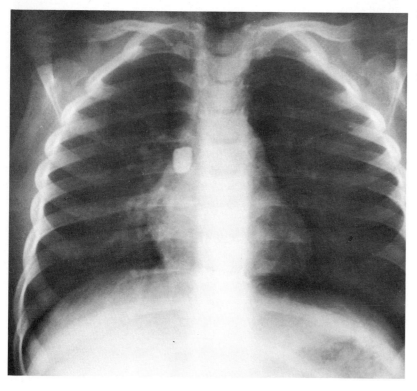

Figure 7. Demosthenes

ANSWER

No, *Demosthenes* was not lucky enough to have swallowed the stone—he aspirated it into his trachea. Note the position of the stone on the lateral chest radiograph (Fig. 8) and then compare this case with the previous one, in which a coin was present in the esophagus.

Removal of the foreign body cured *Demosthenes* of his wish to give further windy speeches.

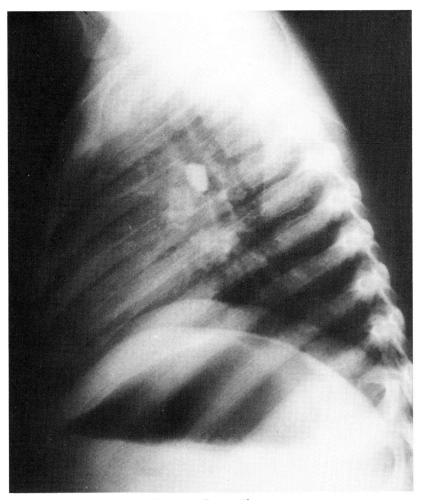

Figure 8. Demosthenes

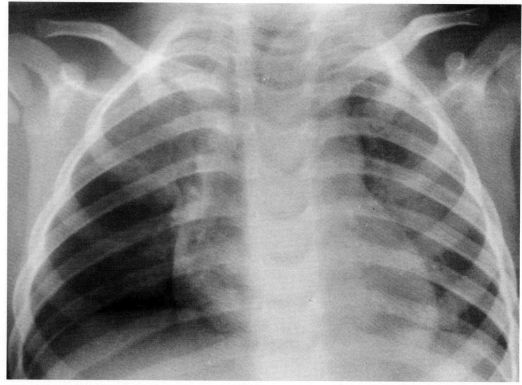

Figure 9.

This young peanut vendor is a 3 year old who enjoyed eating his profits. Unfortunately, coughing and sputtering followed an attempt to gobble down the very last peanut. Where is the profit now?

ANSWER

Note the area of radiolucency demonstrated on the chest radiograph illustrated in Figure 9. The right lower and middle lobes are selectively emphysematous. In this case, our youngster didn't swallow the peanut but aspirated it into the tracheobronchial tree, where it became lodged in the bronchus intermedius. Because of its anatomic orientation, this is a very common site for impaction of airway foreign bodies that create either a total obstruction with ensuing atelectasis or a partial obstruction with a flap or one-way valve mechanism, which leads to air trapping and emphysema.

Foreign bodies in the airway can be very difficult to detect. If an initial inspiratory chest radiograph is normal, a radiograph obtained in expiration may elicit the very helpful finding of air-trapping. Alternatively, radiographs obtained with the patient in the decubitus position may show failure of the obstructed lobe to deflate normally when it is in the dependent position. Finally, fluoroscopic examination of the chest may reveal mediastinal shift. In the normal child the mediastinum remains midline throughout the respiratory cycle. When obstructive emphysema is present, the mediastinum shifts toward the side of the foreign body on inspiration and away from it on expiration.

Bronchoscopy is the procedure of choice to remove the peanut. If the peanut is not removed promptly, bronchial stenosis may result.

TWO CHILDREN WITH RESPIRATORY DISTRESS

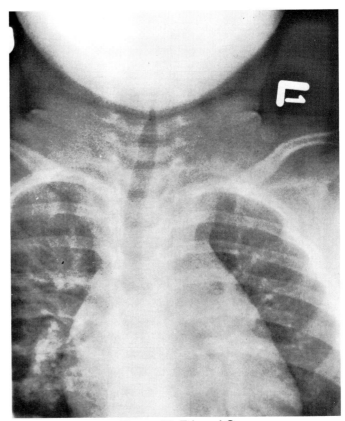

Figure 10. Edward G.

Edward G. is a 3 year old who has had hoarseness and increasing dyspnea for 24 hours. Currently the child has a temperature of 103° F, retraction of the ribs during inspiration, and an inspiratory crow. The boy is not cyanotic, but he seems to have great difficulty breathing, mainly during the inspiratory phase.

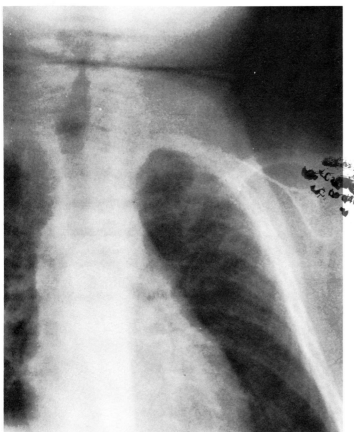

Thomas P., also 3 years old, suddenly had become ill earlier the same day with a sore throat, temperature of 105° F, and severe inspiratory dyspnea. Physical examination shows redness of the posterior oropharynx and surrounding tissues.

You decide that a chest film is indicated and send Thomas P. to the Radiology Department.

Figure 11. Thomas P.

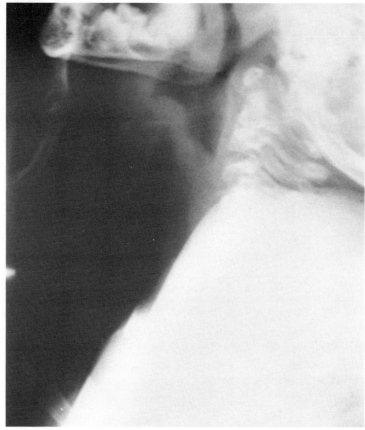

Figure 12. Edward G.

ANSWERS

Edward G. has croup, or laryngotracheobronchitis. Notice the narrowing of the upper trachea caused by edema and inflammation of the area of the trachea just below the vocal cords, the conus elasticus.

Croup is usually caused by a virus and is frequently preceded by a history of an upper respiratory infection. It occurs in children from ages 6 months to 3 years and is usually adequately treated with moist, cool air. Oxygen is added occasionally, but rarely is the disease severe enough to warrant tracheostomy.

This particular child had an additional problem, which is illustrated in Figure 12.

Edward G. became increasingly ill as he was observed in the Emergency Ward. It was difficult to examine him, but the tip of the epiglottis was seen to have a "cherry-red color." Clinically, the condition of the child was deteriorating rapidly with the onset of dysphagia, slight cyanosis, restlessness, and a more "toxic" appearance.

A lateral view of the airway was obtained to evaluate the area that couldn't be seen during physical examination.

What is the diagnosis?

Thomas P. has tonsillitis. The radiograph of his trachea is normal and shows the "square shoulders" of the normal subglottic space. If *Thomas* had been in a good mood, he might have cooperated enough to phonate on command, which would have shown apposition of the true vocal cords, the structures that cast the shadows of the "square shoulders." This technique can be used to demonstrate paralyzed vocal cords.

A specimen was taken for a throat culture, which produced normal flora. He was not treated with antibiotics, and he returned to his normal activity of "beating up" his little sister.

Edward's second film shows the swollen, "thumb-like" appearance of the epiglottis. This is the structure seen above and behind the hyoid bones. It normally has a smooth and slender appearance (see diagram).

Edward has acute epiglottis in addition to his croup. This combination is rather unusual.

Acute epiglottis is commonly a more fulminating condition than croup. The onset of the symptoms is sudden and may progress to respiratory obstruction requiring tracheostomy in a matter of hours. Usually the child complains of intense sore throat and refuses to swallow.

A patient with these symptoms and a fulminating clinical course should have only a limited physical examination of the posterior oropharynx. If the patient is forced to have a thorough examination, this alone may cause obstruction of the airway. Likewise, he should not be forced to lie down for the lateral radiograph of the neck; this, too, may precipitate airway obstruction, and there is no reason why the child should not be sitting in the upright position for the lateral view of the neck.

Treatment will depend upon the degree of respiratory embarrassment. Usually the child is hospitalized so that tracheostomy may be readily performed if necessary. A culture of the epiglottis commonly demonstrates *Haemophilus influenzae*.

In *Edward's* case, simply cool, moist air and antibiotic therapy were sufficient. He did not require a tracheostomy, and after several days in the hospital he was discharged feeling fairly well. His culture grew *Haemophilus influenzae*.

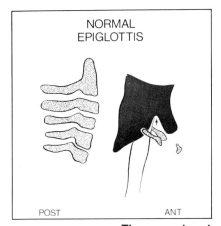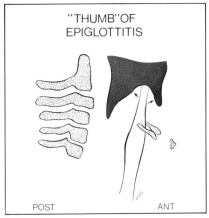

The normal and swollen epiglottis

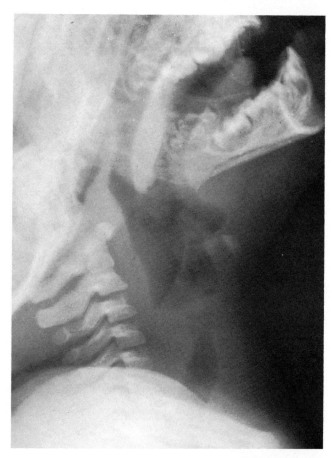

Karen A. is a 9 month old patient who was admitted to the hospital because of suspected aspiration of a tin sailboat.

Figure 13. Karen A.

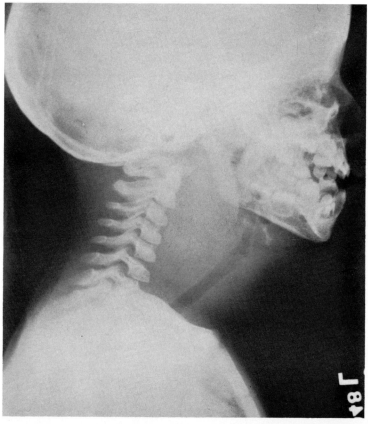

Myrna B. is a 10 month old girl who was quite ill with a temperature of 105.8° F and with difficulty in breathing associated with noisy respiration.

Figure 14. Myrna B.

ANSWERS

Karen A., who was thought to have aspirated a tin sailboat (Fig. 13), was found to have bread crumbs in the trachea. This radiograph was obtained after removal of the bread crumbs and is normal. Notice the slender epiglottis and the horizontal sliver of air beneath the hyoid bone. This is the air in the laryngeal ventricle between the true and false vocal cords.

Compare the width of the tissues anterior to the vertebral bodies in Figure 13 with the same area in Figure 14. *Myrna* has a retropharyngeal abscess. Initially this child had an upper respiratory infection with suppuration of the retropharyngeal lymph nodes. Commonly, dysphagia and dyspnea occur, associated with enlarged cervical lymph nodes and anterior bulging of the posterior pharyngeal wall. Careful fluoroscopy can be used to document thickness of the prevertebral soft tissues. This may be important because expiration, flexion of the neck, and crying will exaggerate *normal* soft tissue thickness. Fluoroscopy during several swallows of barium will help to differentiate the normal retropharyngeal soft tissues from displacement of the esophagus resulting from a retropharyngeal abscess. The treatment includes antibiotic therapy and surgical drainage.

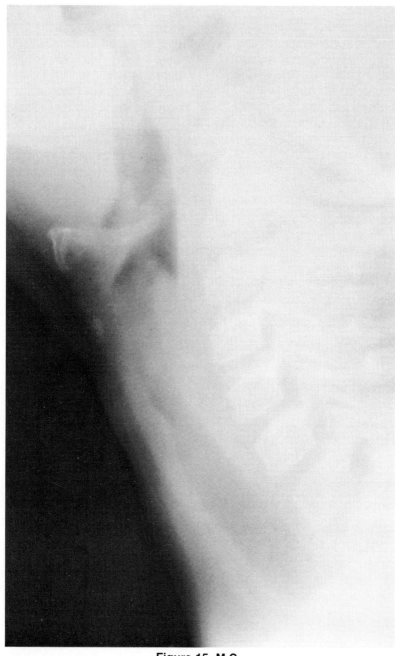

Figure 15. M.C.

M.C., an 8 year old girl, presented with hoarseness, fever, and stridor. Fortunately, she was already in the Emergency Room when she developed dyspnea.

ANSWER

Because of stridor, a lateral radiograph of the neck was obtained. This shows a shaggy, irregular appearance of the tracheal wall that is caused by inspirated material, consisting of mucus and pus that is adherent to the tracheal mucosa. The terms commonly applied to this condition are bacterial tracheitis and membranous croup. The most common organism recovered from culture of the membranes is *Staphylococcus aureus*, although in younger children *Haemophilus influenzae* has been identified.

In addition to appropriate antibiotic therapy, airway maintenance measures such as intubation and tracheostomy may be necessary.

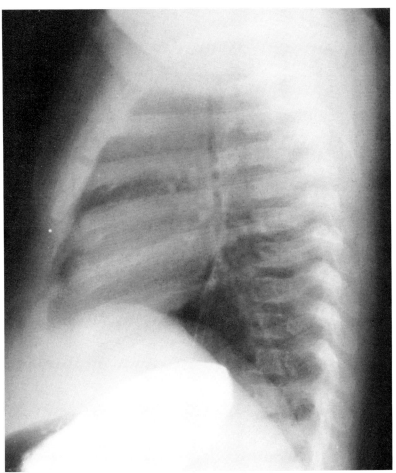

Rasmussen J. Stridor is a 6 month old boy with continuous noisy respiration. Fluoroscopy of the chest confirmed the observation that can be made from the radiographs illustrated in Figure 16. What is your diagnosis?

Figure 16. Rasmussen S.

ANSWER

Rasmussen has stridor, or noisy breathing, which is caused by the abnormal flow of air through a compressed or narrowed portion of the respiratory tract.

The differential diagnosis of stridor includes (1) anomalies of the aorta and pulmonary arteries that cause vascular rings; (2) cysts and other masses of the larynx and trachea; (3) foreign bodies, congenital webs, and stenosis; and (4) inflammatory conditions that cause swelling of the epiglottis (epiglottitis) or subglottic trachea (croup). After all other diagnoses have been excluded, the presence of marked tracheal narrowing on expiration should raise the possibility of tracheomalacia as the cause of the abnormal breathing pattern.

Tracheomalacia is a condition in which tracheal compliance is abnormal, so that collapse or marked narrowing occurs in the intrathoracic trachea during expiration. Be aware, though, that the trachea normally does collapse somewhat during expiration and that the diagnosis of tracheomalacia is therefore based on the degree of narrowing.

The child with tracheomalacia usually outgrows the condition but may need extra special care during bouts of upper respiratory infection.

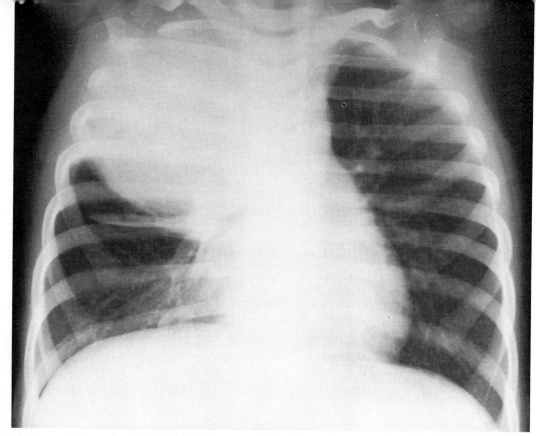

Figure 17. Tammy G.

Tammy G., a 3 year old girl, is brought to the hospital with a history of repeated colds.

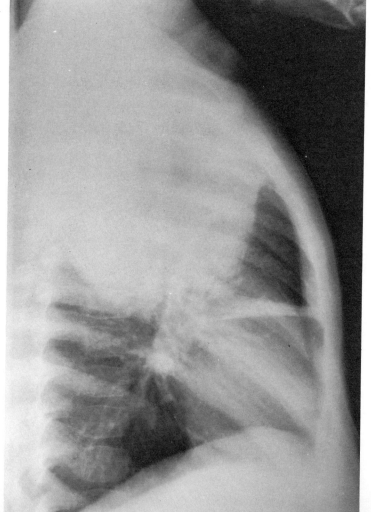

Figure 18. Tammy G.

ANSWER

Tammy G. has virtually no symptoms. Her mother noticed that it took longer for her to "throw off a cold" than for her brothers and sister. Imagine everyone's surprise when the chest radiograph revealed the huge mass that we see in Figures 17 and 18. There are several clues involved in the correct interpretation of these radiographs, and they must all be utilized in order to arrive at a reasonable differential diagnosis of this lesion.

In the first place, it would be helpful to decide whether this mass is more likely to be in the lung or in the mediastinum. Notice that on the lateral view, the anterior lung-mass interface makes an acute angle with the sternum. This usually suggests that the mass is extrapleural, compressing normal lung tissue and causing the plate-like atelectasis seen just beneath the mass against the minor fissure. If this *is* a mediastinal mass, localization into the proper compartment of the mediastinum should lead to a differential diagnosis that includes certain possibilities and makes other conditions less likely.

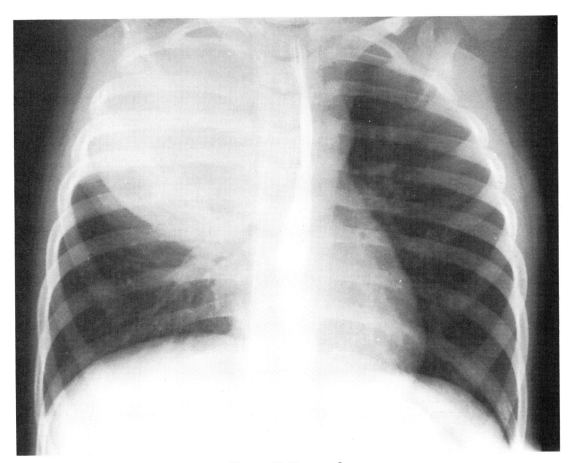

Figure 19. Tammy G.

Note that in Figure 19 the barium opacified esophagus is deviated to the left (the patient's left). Since the esophagus is a posterior mediastinal structure, this mass at least extends into the posterior mediastinum and may originate there. The most common masses arising in the posterior mediastinum are neurogenic tumors.

Now observe in Figure 20 the erosion of the posterior portion of the second rib and widening of the second intercostal space. This tells you that this mass has developed slowly, because it takes time for such a rib deformity to develop. So, this is a mass lesion, probably arising in the posterior mediastinum. It has been present for a long time and probably is a tumor of neurogenic origin.

This little girl had a thoracotomy and resection of the mass. It was, indeed, an extrapleural posterior mediastinal mass that proved to be a ganglioneuroma. These are tumors that arise from the spinal nerves and can invade the spinal canal; thus, any evidence of destruction of the vertebrae or pedicles (or symptoms or physical findings of spinal cord involvement) is an indication for a myelogram or contrast-enhanced computed tomography. In this case there was no spinal cord involvement, and since surgery this child has had an uncomplicated recovery.

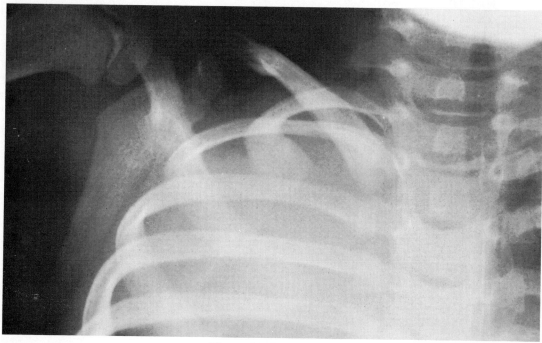

Figure 20. Tammy G.

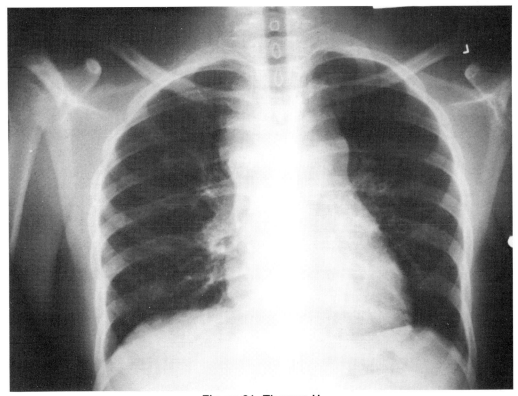

Figure 21. Thomas H.

Thomas H., a 16 year old boy, was seen by his family doctor because of night sweats and weight loss.

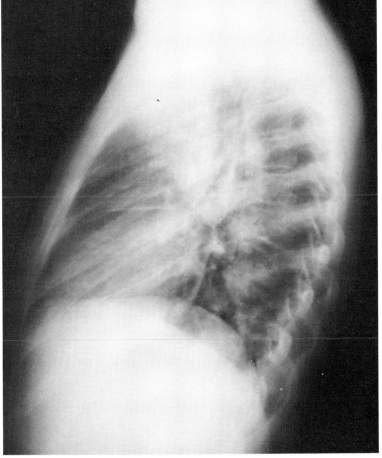

Figure 22. Thomas H.

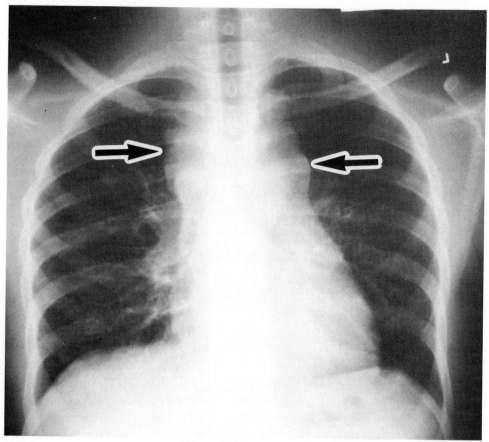

Figure 23. Thomas H.

ANSWER

The key to correct interpretation of *Thomas'* frontal radiograph is recognition of the widened mediastinum (arrows, Fig. 23). On the lateral view, a mass is present anteriorly. (This was even better demonstrated by computed tomography [Figs. 24 and 25].)

We have already discussed posterior mediastinal masses (see page 18). In children, 30 per cent of mediastinal masses are found in the middle mediastinum, and the most likely causes are foregut duplication, bronchogenic cysts, and lymphadenopathy. Anterior mediastinal masses also make up 30 per cent of mediastinal masses seen in children. Lymphoma, thymic masses, and teratoma are the common causes, while thyroid masses are relatively uncommon in children.

Thomas H. has Hodgkin's disease, and the mediastinal mass present in his chest radiograph is caused by lymphadenopathy.

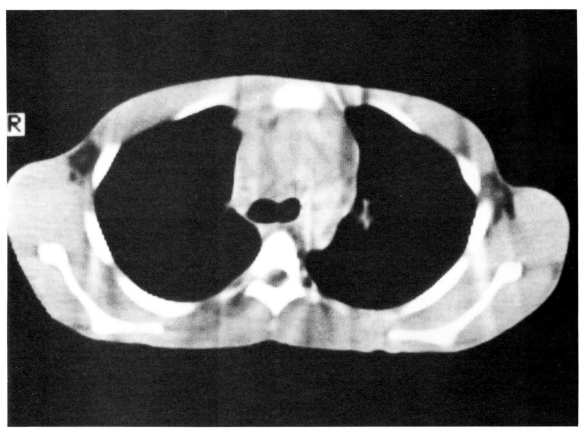

Figure 24. Thomas H.

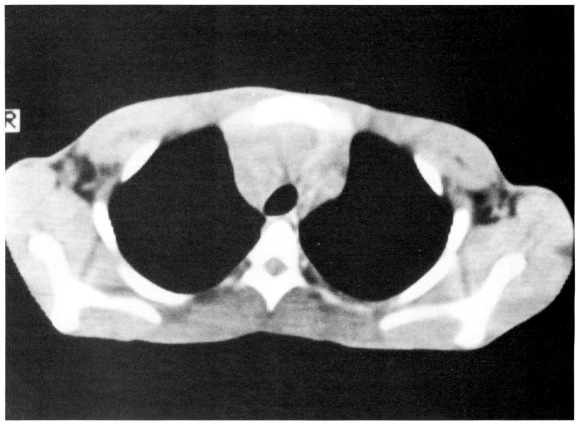

Figure 25. Thomas H.

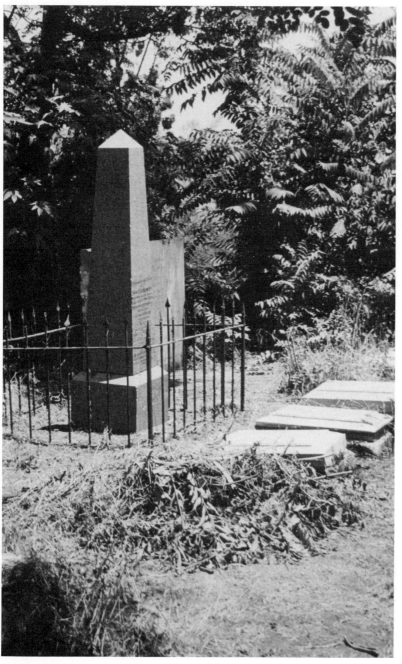

Hodgkin's disease was described without benefit of x-ray by Thomas Hodgkin. Do you know what Hodgkin died of and where he was buried? (Photograph courtesy of Prof. Schwartz and Prof. J. Labowitz.)

Figure 26.

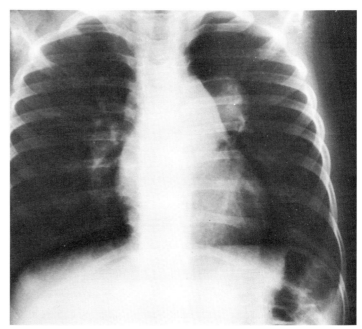

Figure 27. Irene H.

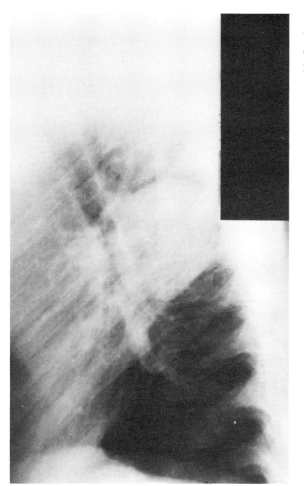

Figure 28. Irene H.

Irene Hochberg is a 6 year old girl whose chest radiograph was obtained because of persistent paroxysmal coughing.

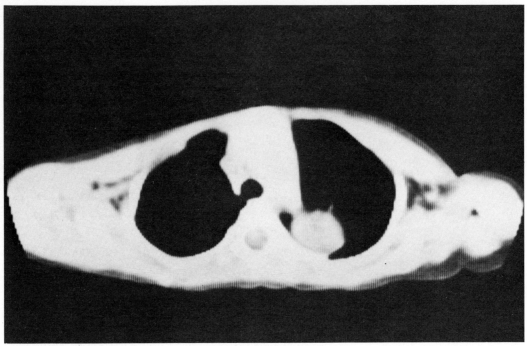

Figure 29. Irene H.

ANSWER

The frontal and lateral chest radiographs (Figs. 27 and 28) and x-ray computed tomographic study (Fig. 29) show a mass originating in the middle mediastinum and extending into the posterior mediastinum. No calcification or fat is seen, and the margins of the mass are smooth.

Irene's mediastinal mass was removed at surgery and proved to be a bronchogenic cyst. However, there are no radiologic criteria whereby this could be distinguished from a foregut duplication. Removal of a bronchogenic cyst is necessary, as it may displace and compress normal mediastinal structures. If such displacement and compression occur and a bronchus is obstructed, respiratory symptoms may result. In *Irene's* case, though, the coughing was produced by good old-fashioned sinusitis and postnasal drip.

Pandora B. was seen by her pediatrician because of fever. Although the doctor did not suspect pneumonia, *Pandora's* mother insisted on a chest x-ray because a third cousin, four times removed, had just recovered from "double walking pneumonia."

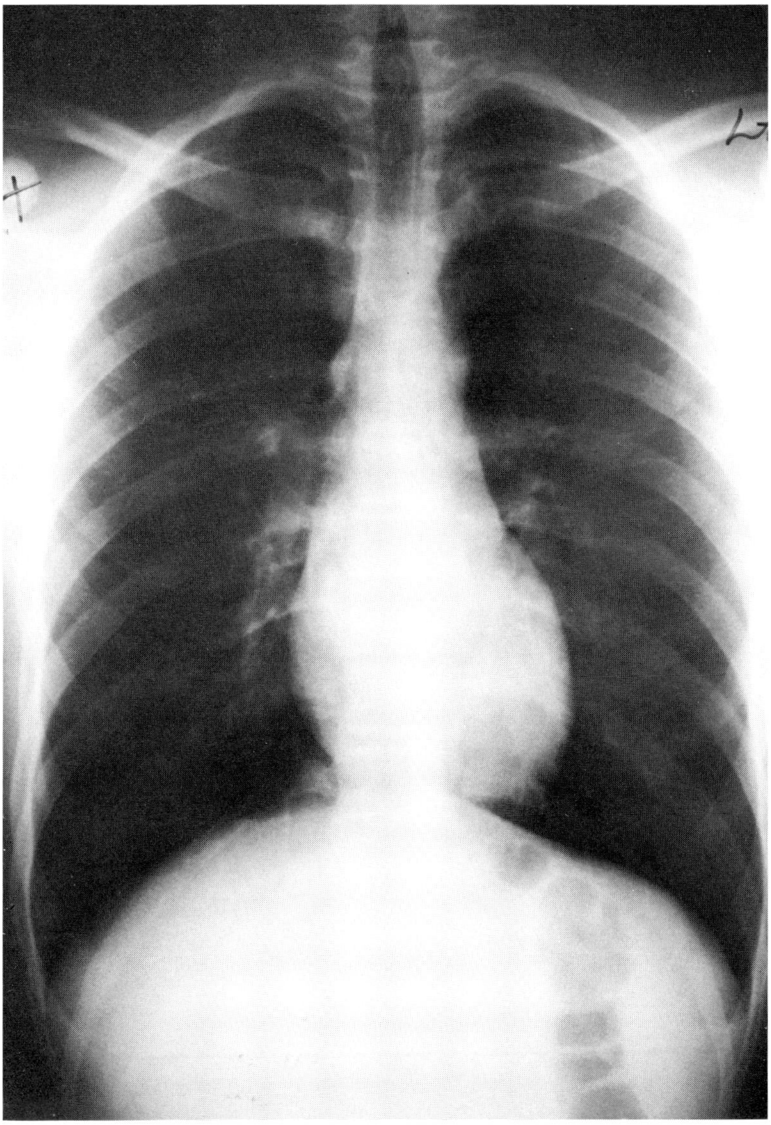

Figure 30. Pandora B.

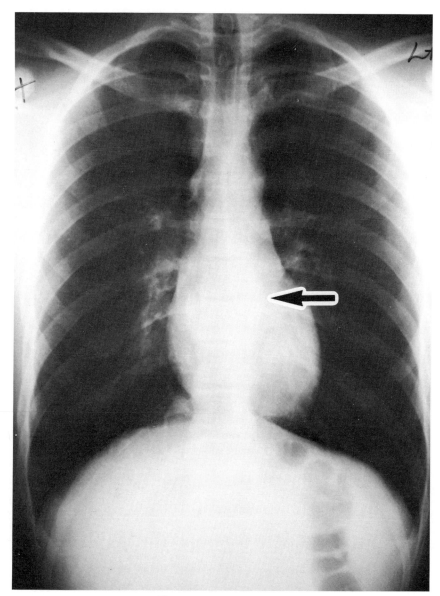

Figure 31. Pandora B.

ANSWER

Sometimes mediastinal lesions are expanding space-occupying masses that are accompanied by clinical symptoms such as chest pain, cough, hemoptysis, or dysphagia. On many occasions, however, as with *Pandora*, they are recognized as incidental findings on radiographs obtained for other reasons.

In Figure 30, did you notice the bump adjacent to the tenth vertebral body? This shadow is definitely abnormal (Fig. 31).

An x-ray computed tomographic scan (Fig. 32) confirms the presence of a mass, which is adjacent to the aorta (arrow) and has a smooth border. This lesion was removed surgically and was found to be a foregut duplication cyst. Such cysts may be lined by any type of alimentary tract epithelium and expand as secretions accumulate. Since some such cysts communicate with the alimentary tract, they occasionally may contain gas.

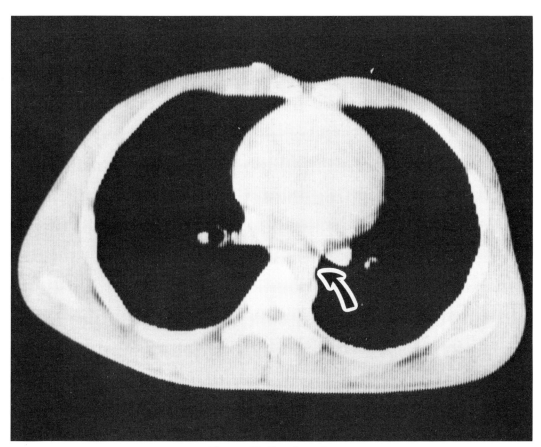

Figure 32. Pandora B.

THREE CHILDREN SENT TO RADIOLOGY FOR EVALUATION OF "URI's"

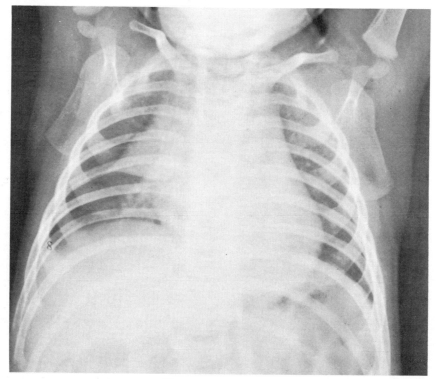

Figure 33. Shadrach

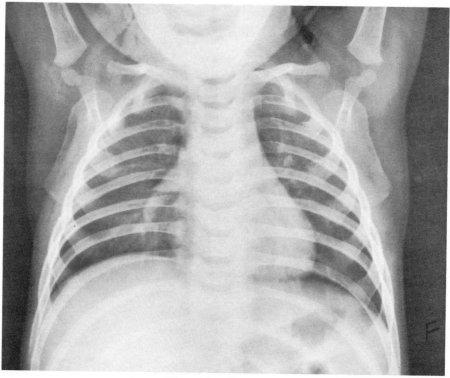

Figure 34. Meshach

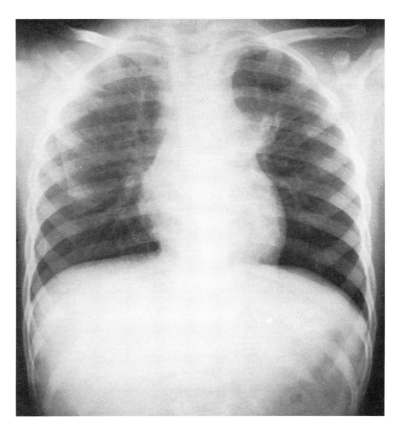

Figure 35. Abednego

Here are three patients named **Shadrach** (Fig. 33), **Meshach** (Fig. 34), and **Abednego** (Figs. 35 and 36). They all have "URI's," or upper respiratory infections. Chest radiographs are being performed to rule out pneumonia.

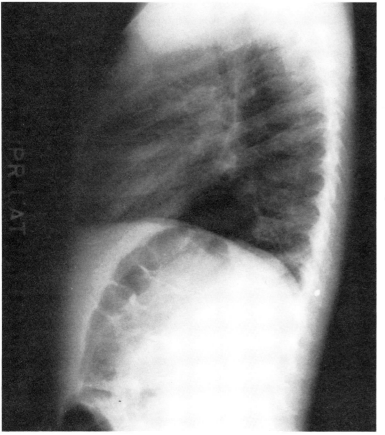

Figure 36. Abednego

ANSWERS

Shadrach and *Meshach* are the same patient, an 18 month old boy examined because of suspected upper respiratory infection. Why does the mediastinum appear wider in *Shadrach*, and what about the mass extending into the right lung field?

This is the appearance of the normal thymus gland on an expiratory radiograph. Note that you can only count eight ribs posteriorly. Now look at *Meshach's* radiograph. It was made 30 seconds later but was taken during inspiration and shows nine ribs posteriorly. On this radiograph, the thymus appears much smaller and is seen overlying the right main pulmonary artery.

Figure 33 was obtained during expiration and demonstrates the "thymic sail sign." This is the projection of the *normal* thymus into the minor fissure of the right lung. Sometimes indentation upon the thymus by the anterior ribs or costal cartilage creates a rippled appearance that has been termed the "thymic wave sign."

Abednego's chest films (Figs. 35 and 36) show a prominent left hilus with a streaky infiltrate radiating into the left upper lobe. On the lateral film there is a fullness of the hilar region, suggesting that the infiltrate in the left upper lobe is accompanied by enlargement of hilar lymph nodes.

This complex of findings should suggest the possibility of primary tuberculosis. Such a child usually has only non-specific symptoms such as cough, fever, and sometimes weight loss and lethargy. The radiographic features of primary tuberculosis include the pulmonary infiltrate, enlarged hilar nodes, and lymphangitic streaks that may be seen extending from the enlarged hilar nodes to the pulmonary infiltrate. These features are termed "the primary complex." Although reinfection tuberculosis in adults affects mainly the upper lobes, primary tuberculosis may affect any lobe.

The diagnosis is established on the basis of a positive skin test, the chest radiograph, and, hopefully, bacteriologic confirmation.

Although in most children the pulmonary lesion of primary tuberculosis will heal spontaneously, in a few cases miliary tuberculosis, pleural effusion, and, most importantly, meningitis will develop. Meningitis is the most common cause of death in children with pulmonary tuberculosis.

Abednego's condition was recognized promptly as pulmonary tuberculosis, and treatment was begun. Unfortunately, the home situation was very bad, a "diagnosis" you established when you saw the two shotgun pellets, one in the back and one in the abdomen. The circumstances surrounding these injuries were not clear, but it was known that several months after these radiographs were made, the child fired a revolver at his mother. The child was removed to another state by the family, and no follow-up was possible.

Other Pitfalls to Avoid

Decide which statements are true:

This 2 year old boy (Fig. 37) has

- A. Pneumonia
- B. Cardiomegaly
- C. Both of the above
- D. None of the above
- E. Can't tell

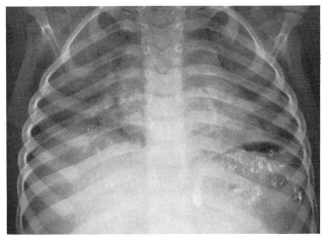

Figure 37.

This 2 year old boy (Fig. 38) has

- A. Pneumonia
- B. Cardiomegaly
- C. Is the same patient shown in Figure 37.

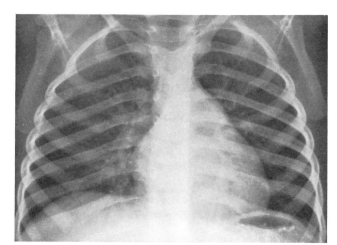

Figure 38.

ANSWERS

If you said Figure 37 demonstrated cardiomegaly and pneumonia, you failed to take into account the phase of respiration. There are seven posterior ribs seen on the right side at the level of the diaphragm. This has resulted in crowding of the bronchovascular shadows in the lower lobes, creating the appearance of pneumonia. Note also that the heart has a more transverse position than in Figure 38. This is also a reflection of the poor inspiration and resulting high level of the diaphragm.

In Figure 38 there are nine posterior ribs seen at the level of the right hemidiaphragm. The lungs are clear, and the heart appears normal. This radiograph was made during inspiration just a few seconds after the previous radiograph on the same patient.

Before you evaluate a child for cardiomegaly, pneumonia, or even congestive failure, you must insist that the level of the right hemidiaphragm be at the ninth or tenth posterior rib in order to be certain that he has taken an adequate inspiration.

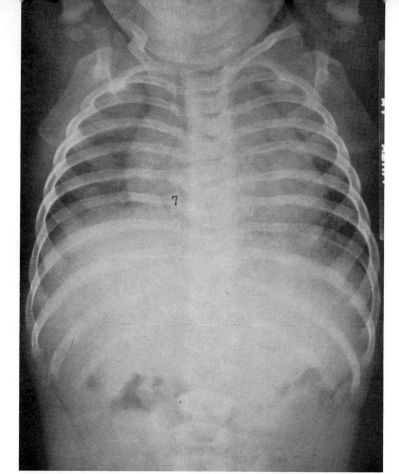

Figure 39.

Figure 40.

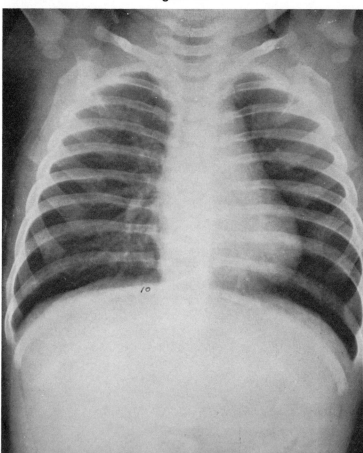

This child's heart is enlarged (Fig. 39):

A. True

B. False

C. This is a stupid question.

ANSWER: C.

You can't accurately determine cardiac size from an expiratory radiograph. The level of the right hemidiaphragm is at the seventh posterior rib.

An adequate inspiratory radiograph (Fig. 40) shows clearly that the heart is normal in size. If the level of the diaphragm is between the ninth and tenth posterior ribs, the inspiratory effort is adequate, and the heart size can be evaluated.

In time, you will count ribs only occasionally because your brain will have learned to judge lung volume without this step.

This baby has significant shift of the mediastinum accompanied by a difference in radiodensity of the right and left lungs (Fig. 41):

A. True

B. False

C. This is like the question on the opposite page—it's stupid.

ANSWER: C.

This baby is rotated toward his right, creating the appearance of a mediastinal shift and differential aeration of the lungs. Figure 42 is a straight radiograph, and all is well with the world—no mediastinal shift and normal-appearing lungs. So how can you tell if a radiograph is rotated? You look at the clavicles to see if they are symmetrical, and you look at the anterior ribs to determine whether you can see as much of the anterior ribs on one side as on the other.

(On the right side there are pleural and rib changes caused by previous surgery for tetralogy of Fallot.)

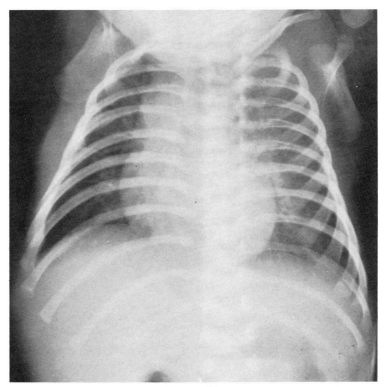

Figure 41.

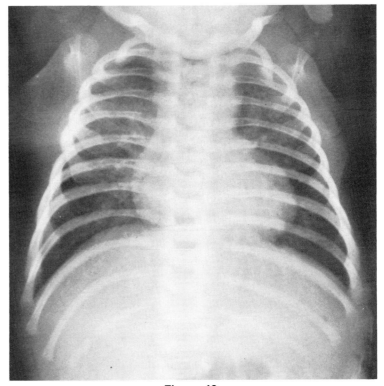

Figure 42.

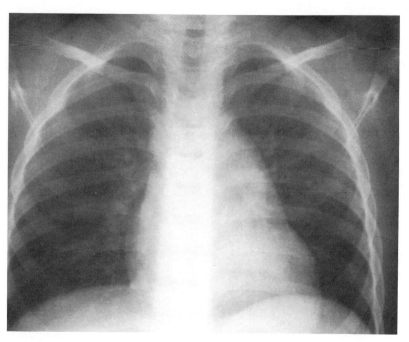

5 a.m.　　　　　　**7-9**

Figure 43. Jupiter K.

Jupiter Kozlowsky is a 7 year old boy with fever and cough who was seen in the Emergency Room and sent home with an expectorant.

ANSWER

If you assumed we wouldn't show you a normal chest radiograph, think again. We just did!

However, *Jupiter* got worse, and his parents brought him to the Emergency Room again. A new radiograph was obtained and is illustrated in Figure 44. What is your opinion now?

The density present behind the heart is called a "round pneumonia." Round pneumonias are usually of bacterial eti-ology and tend to arise in the lower lobes—the dependent parts of the lungs. This mass-like density results from rapid expansion of pulmonary consolidation in a concentric fashion. The radiologic change that occurred in *Jupiter's* case happened over a 12 hour period. Previous normal chest radiographs or normal radiographs obtained after recovery help to exclude pathologic conditions other than pneumonia.

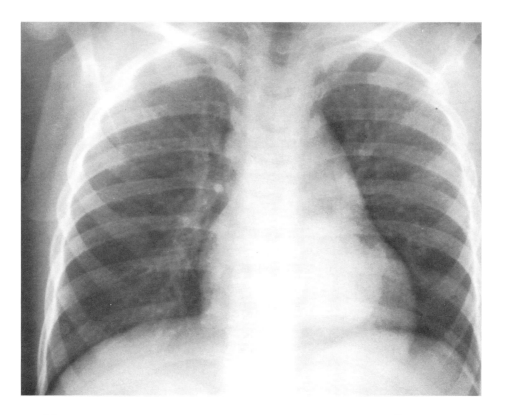

5 p.m.   7-9

Figure 44. Jupiter K.

COUGH, FEVER, AND RAPID RESPIRATION AND PULSE IN A THREE MONTH OLD BABY

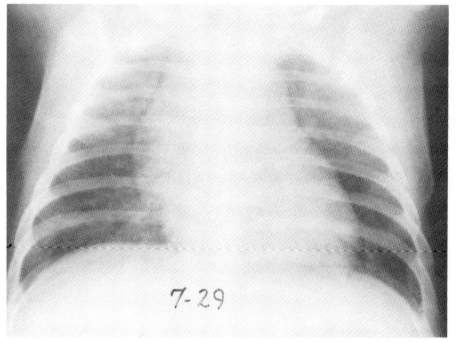

Figure 45. Kenneth M.

On July 29, **Kenneth M.** was brought to the Outpatient Clinic by his mother, who stated that *Kenneth* was irritable, cried a lot, and had a temperature of 103° F rectally. He also coughed so much that he couldn't sleep.

The physical examination confirmed the elevation of the temperature and showed the pulse to be 130 beats per minute and the rate of respiration to be 50 breaths per minute. Examination of the chest revealed wheezing but no rales.

The chest x-ray on July 29 was negative (Fig. 45). *Kenneth* was treated symptomatically.

He returned on August 21 with a recurrence of the same symptoms. How would you report this chest study (Fig. 46)?

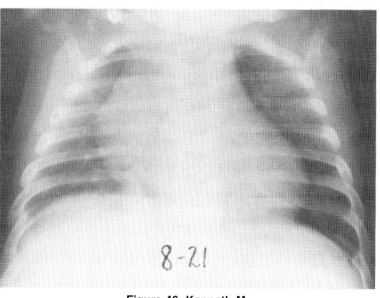

Figure 46. Kenneth M.

ANSWER

The chest radiograph of August 21 has changed; there are two very significant new findings. The early study showed no fluid in the pleural space and no definite consolidation in the lungs. The August 21 film shows obliteration of the right costophrenic sulcus and a small amount of fluid along the right chest wall. This is accompanied by consolidation in a portion of the right lower lobe, close to the heart.

The findings of fluid in the pleural space associated with consolidation in the lung should suggest staphylococcal pneumonia. Usually the radiologist can't predict the bacterial cause in a given case (a fact the radiologist *and* clinician frequently forget). However, staphylococcal pneumonia is often an exception. The involvement is unilateral about 80 per cent of the time. The pneumonia is not commonly accompanied by mediastinal lymph node enlargement. Pleural involvement is seen in 90 per cent of the cases, and pneumothorax and pyopneumothorax occur in one fourth of the cases.

By 11:00 P.M. on August 23, *Kenneth* had formed a small cyst (pneumatocele) just medial to the gross amount of fluid now present in the right pleural space (Fig. 47). (This baby has been filmed in the supine position.) In most or all instances, a pneumatocele represents a subpleural air collection. Necrosis of a portion of a bronchiolar wall permits air to dissect the interstitial pulmonary tissues, where it forms a tract to the subpleural space. It may occur in a matter of hours, and there may be coalescence of pneumatoceles. It may take months for these cavities to clear.

Is there a differential diagnosis for unilateral consolidation with pleural reaction? Yes; in primary tuberculous pneumonia and, rarely, in pneumococcal pneumonia and *Haemophilus influenzae* pneumonia, similar findings may occur. However, the additional finding of a pneumatocele is highly suggestive that the causative organism is *Staphylococcus*.

In *Kenneth's* case, the diagnosis was suggested by the radiograph. Cultures were taken and treatment was initiated on the presumption that this was staphylococcal pneumonia. The cultures of the blood and pleural fluid established that this diagnosis was correct. The child recovered.

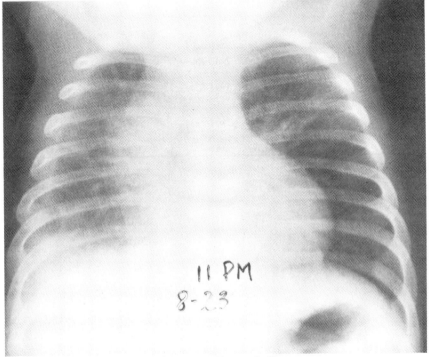

Figure 47. Kenneth M.

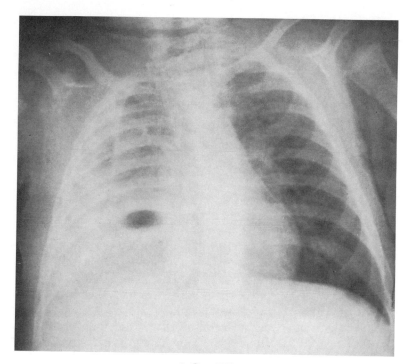

12-7

Figure 48.

This is another ex-
ample of pneumatocele
formation in staphylo-
coccal pneumonia.

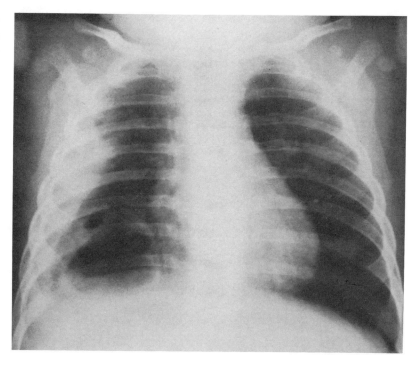

12-21

Figure 49.

In Figures 48 and 49, a thin-walled cavity called a pneumatocele is located in the right lower lobe. Infiltrate surrounds the pneumatocele, and on the second radiograph (Fig. 49) an air-fluid level is present. This indicates communication between the pneumatocele and the airways, with accumulation of inflammatory products in the cyst-like lesion. Air may become trapped within a pneumatocele, resulting sometimes in a dramatic expansion of the lesion (Fig. 50). With antibiotic therapy and time, the pneumatocele will gradually resolve.

You should know that another common association of pneumatocele formation in children is the chemical pneumonitis that results from accidental hydrocarbon ingestion.

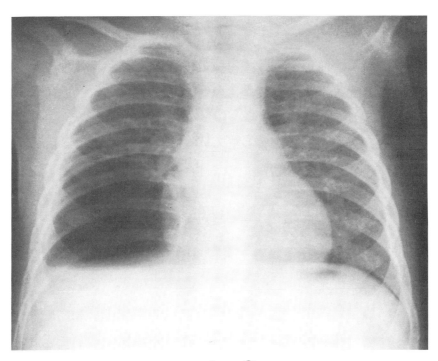

4-2

Figure 50.

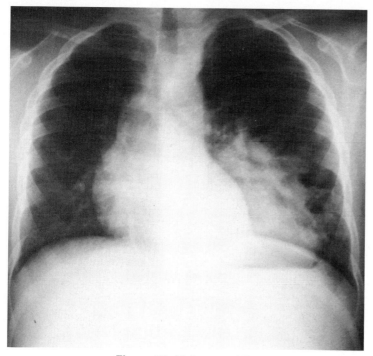

Figure 51. Mohammed D.

Mohammad D. is a 7 year old boy who has had repeated respiratory tract infections for many years. During one of his febrile episodes, these radiographs were obtained. What are the crucial observations? What would you do next?

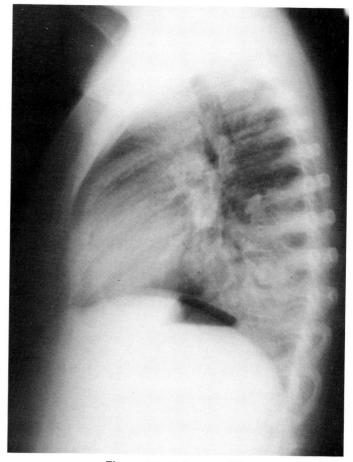

Figure 52. Mohammed D.

Note that on the frontal radiograph a triangular-shaped density is present within the left lower lobe. There are also associated air-fluid levels, which are indicative of infection. (Given *Mohammed's* history, does a diagnosis come to mind?) The next study performed on our patient was a bronchogram (Fig. 52A), which demonstrates no communication between the tracheobronchial tree and this lesion. Instead, the bronchi were splayed around the density.

The final diagnostic study performed on *Mohammed* was an aortogram (Fig. 53). It shows that the affected portion of the lung is supplied by systemic rather than by pulmonary arteries. Because of the typical location and radiographic appearance, the diagnosis of an infected pulmonary sequestration was made.

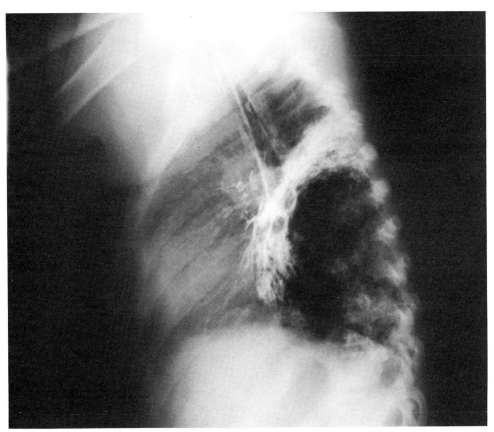

Figure 52A. Mohammed D.

A pulmonary sequestration represents nonfunctional pulmonary tissue. It does not communicate with the bronchial tree and is perfused by systemic arterial supply from the aorta. There are two types of sequestration, and *Mohammed* has the common intrapulmonary type rather than the uncommon extrapulmonary type. Children with this disorder frequently come to their physicians because of recurrent pneumonia. In the case of extralobar sequestrations, these patients are frequently asymptomatic, and their problem is often detected when a chest radiograph shows an intrathoracic mass. In both types of sequestration the treatment is surgical removal of the abnormal pulmonary tissue.

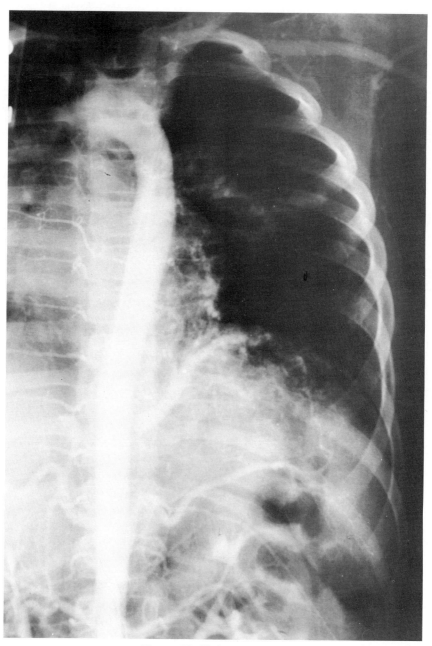

Figure 53. Mohammed D.

COUGH PRODUCTIVE OF FOUL SPUTUM

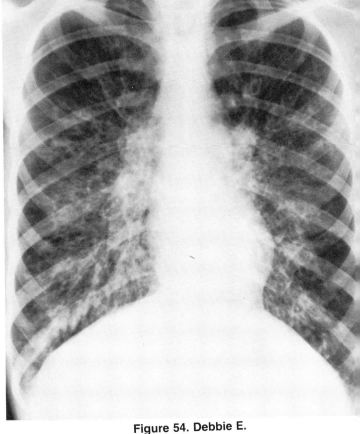

Figure 54. Debbie E.

Debbie E. is a 12 year old girl who is an old friend of the hospital (she has two hospital charts—both thicker than the Manhattan telephone directory). She returned to the Chest Clinic complaining of producing increasing amounts of foul-smelling sputum associated with decreasing ability to keep up with her friends when they played games that involved any type of exercise.

Debbie is a thin 12 year old, much shorter than her classmates in school. Her chest has a very emphysematous configuration. At examination, her vital signs show an increased respiratory rate for her (about 24 breaths per minute) and a temperature of 99.6° F orally. Auscultation of the chest reveals bilateral moist rales.

The diagnosis of *Debbie's* chronic condition can be made from the chest PA and lateral views (Figs. 54 and 55), although in *Debbie's* case the diagnosis was established when she was a baby.

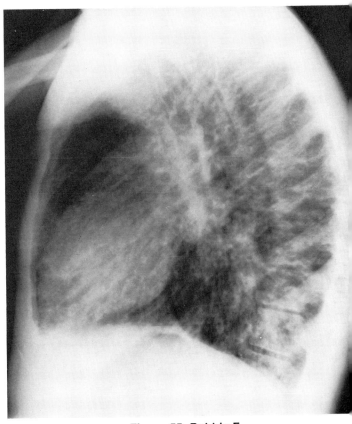

Figure 55. Debbie E.

ANSWER

Debbie has cystic fibrosis, a disease of the exocrine glands, which is inherited as an autosomal recessive trait. It involves the pancreas, mucous glands of the bronchi, and salivary and sweat glands. The characteristic secretion of the affected glands is a thick mucus that plugs the ducts.

In the lungs the thick mucus causes occlusion of bronchi and resulting atelectasis. Peribronchial inflammation occurs, and the bronchial walls become thickened or "cuffed." Air-trapping also occurs and is manifested clinically and radiologically as overinflation. There is a wide AP diameter to the chest, as seen on the lateral view. This is accompanied by the low level of the diaphragm, causing the heart to appear small.

The occlusion of exocrine glands in the pancreas causes atrophy of the parenchyma and results in reduced enzyme secretion and malabsorption. In the newborn, the meconium may be so thick that bowel obstruction occurs. If the meconium leaks into the peritoneal cavity, there is prompt calcification, indicating meconium peritonitis. Obstruction of the bile ducts may lead to biliary cirrhosis, and these children may have gastrointestinal bleeding from esophageal varices.

Other associated conditions include nasal polyps that fill the nasal cavity. Sometimes rectal prolapse occurs.

In *Debbie's* case, the pulmonary manifestations are not yet disabling. She has frequent respiratory infections, but appropriate antibiotics and "respiratory toilet" (postural drainage and chest thumping to mobilize secretions) enable her to handle the infections fairly well. The other manifestations of cystic fibrosis do not appear to have affected her clinically.

The diagnosis of cystic fibrosis in children can usually be suspected if emphysema, chronic lung changes, and peribronchial cuffing (better illustrated in a later case) are present together on the radiograph.

In the older child with cystic fibrosis, the viscosity of the feces can lead to intussusception, as illustrated in Figure 56.

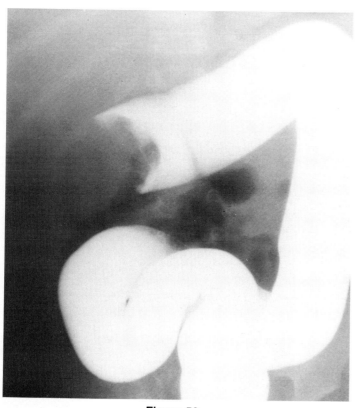

Figure 56.

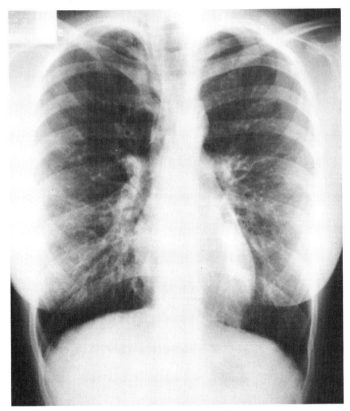

Figure 57. Kathy C.

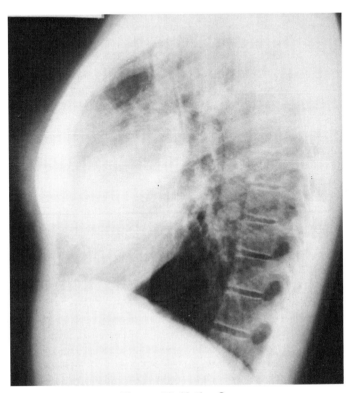

These frontal and lateral chest radiographs were obtained on **Kathy Clark,** a 16 year old known asthmatic, who had an "attack" during a school dance. What do you see?

Figure 58. Kathy C.

ANSWER

Did you notice on the lateral chest radiograph the radiolucencies outlining the great vessels and the anterior trachea? These findings are the hallmark of pneumomediastinum. During *Kathy's* asthmatic attack, air has dissected from the alveoli into the lung interstitium and then into the mediastinum. A pneumomediastinum is important to recognize because it may precede the development of a pneumothorax, a potentially life-threatening complication. The air can also extend into the neck and other soft tissues and be manifested as subcutaneous emphysema.

The frontal radiograph of the chest shows hyperexpansion of the lungs, a roentgen manifestation of reactive airway disease.

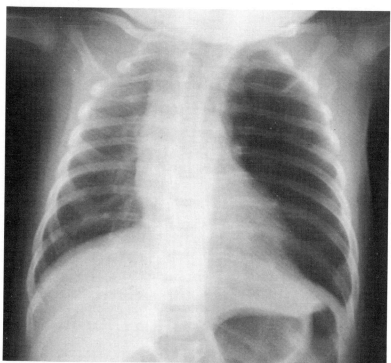

Baby girl **Zinfandel** developed progressive respiratory distress shortly after birth. This radiograph provides significant information as to the cause of the problem. What is your opinion?

Figure 59. B. Girl Zinfandel

ANSWER

Baby Girl Zinfandel's chest radiograph shows a hyperlucent, hyperexpanded left upper lobe and a collapsed left lower lobe. This x-ray is highly suggestive of a condition that can be a surgical emergency and that is known as congenital lobar emphysema. The upper lobes, right middle lobe, and lingula are the commonly involved lobes. The overdistention is felt to be caused by abnormal function and structure of the bronchus such that normal deflation cannot occur on expiration. This in turn causes compression atelectasis of the neighboring lobes. Because the condition is usually progressive in terms of respiratory distress and emphysema, prompt surgical therapy is usually imperative.

THREE NEWBORNS WITH RESPIRATORY DISTRESS

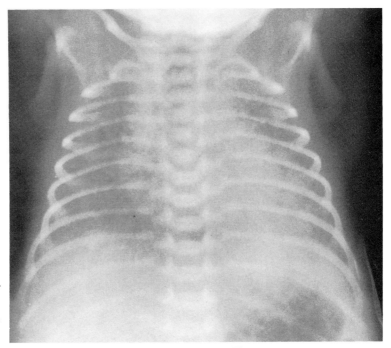

Baby Boy Lucifer (Fig. 60) is a 1900 gram premature newborn who developed rapid respiration, grunting, and retraction of the intercostal spaces approximately one-half hour after birth.

Figure 60. Lucifer

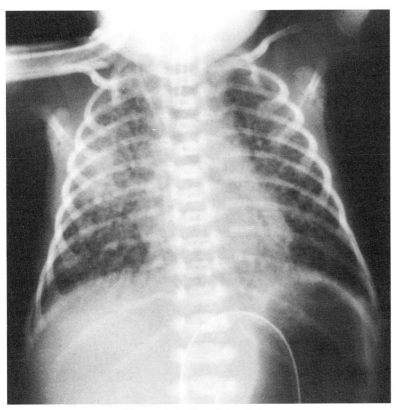

Figure 61. Mephistopheles

Baby Boy Mephistopheles (Fig. 61) is also premature. This radiograph was taken at 9 hours of age shortly after intubation, which was done because of increasing respiratory distress and cyanosis.

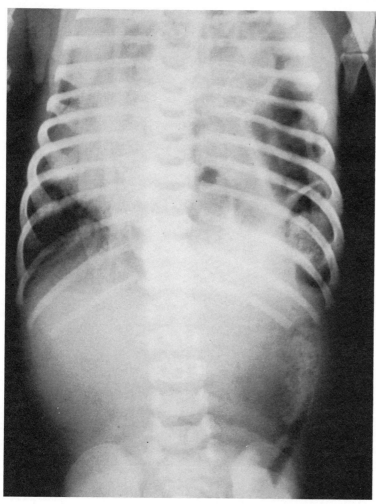

Figure 62. Beelzebub

Baby Boy Beelzebub (Fig. 62) was 2 weeks old at the time this radiograph was obtained. He appeared normal for the first seven days and then developed difficulty in breathing while nursing. The physical examination showed that the cardiac apex was shifted to the right, and gurgling sounds were heard on the left side of the chest.

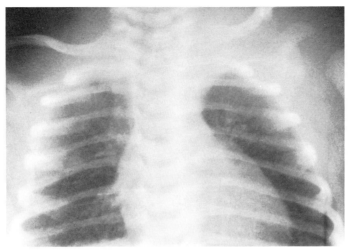

Figure 63. Normal newborn lungs for comparison

ANSWERS

Baby Boy Lucifer and *Baby Boy Mephistopheles* both have lungs that are not normally ventilated. If you look closely at *Baby Boy Lucifer's* radiograph, you will see radiolucent strips that radiate from the hili (air bronchograms). The generic term applied to his lungs is "underventilated," or "atelectatic." Many of the alveoli are collapsed; in severe cases, almost all the alveoli are airless. The bronchioles, alveolar ducts, and occasional alveoli are overdistended.

Such babies have severe hyaline membrane disease. This condition is usually seen only in premature babies. Clinically, shortly after birth they develop tachypnea, grunting, retraction of the intercostal spaces, and cyanosis.

The pathologic basis for the radiographic features are the "hyaline membranes," which are largely composed of fibrin and are derived from the blood in the infant's pulmonary capillaries. The fibrin deposits cause a decrease in lung compliance, and respiratory distress results.

The widespread atelectasis is caused by reduced amounts of surfactant. This substance decreases the surface tension in the alveoli; without it, the alveoli collapse on expiration. The granular (or reticulonodular) appearance of the lungs is caused by discrete areas of hyperinflation surrounded by atelectatic foci. This also causes the "air bronchogram" effect.

Complications of this condition include pneumothorax, pneumomediastinum, and pulmonary interstitial emphysema. Pulmonary interstitial emphysema occurs when air dissects into the lung interstitium because of high respiratory pressures. This creates the reticular lucent pattern seen in Figure 61, *Baby Boy Mephistopheles'* radiograph. Air can then extend into the mediastinum and rupture into the pleura to create a pneumothorax.

Baby Boy Beelzebub's radiograph (Fig. 62) shows peculiar gas-containing structures superimposed on the left lung. As a matter of fact, little bowel gas is

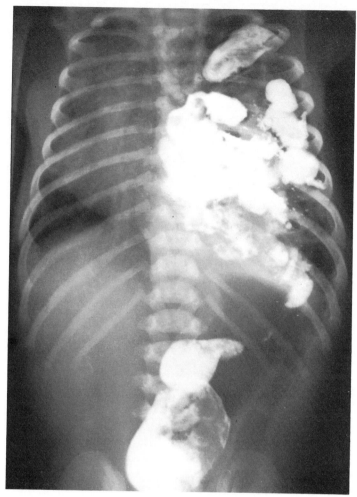

Figure 64. Beelzebub

seen in the abdomen. This should lead you to suspect that the bowel contents have herniated into the chest and that these structures are dilated gas-filled loops of intestine. You had already suspected this because physical examination revealed gurgling sounds in the child's chest.

Figure 64 shows the barium study performed to prove the diagnosis. This is an older case; today a barium study would not have been done because the plain films establish the diagnosis.

This patient had a diaphragmatic hernia through the foramen of Bochdalek. It usually occurs on the left side (maybe because the liver inhibits its occurrence on the right side). The hernia may involve the liver, kidney, spleen, stomach, small bowel, or colon.

Immediately after the diagnosis was made, surgery was performed, and the abdominal contents were replaced. *Baby Boy Beelzebub* had an uncomplicated recovery.

(By the way, did you notice that the "normal newborn" (Fig. 63) has a fractured left clavicle?)

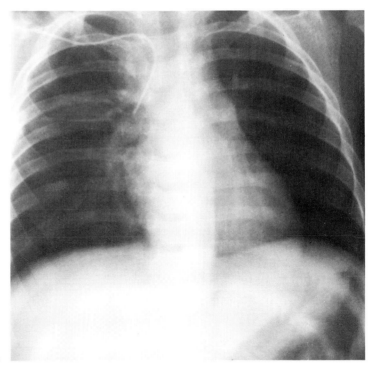

Figure 65. Shirley W.

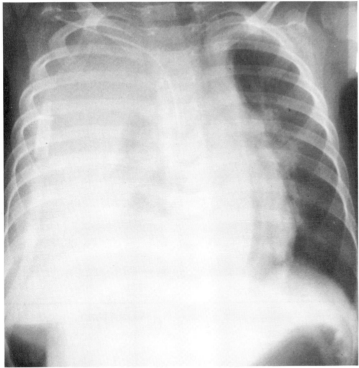

Figure 66. Shirley W.

The radiograph on the left (Fig. 65) was obtained on a 2 year old girl, **Shirley Waters,** after placement of a central venous line. The house officer in charge could not withdraw blood into the line, but he had nevertheless proceeded with administration of total parenteral nutrition (TPN) fluid. Because Patient *Waters* developed tachypnea and respiratory distress, the radiograph illustrated in Figure 66 was obtained the following day.

What is your diagnosis, and what could you have done to address the problem after you examined the first radiograph?

ANSWER

Let's begin with Figure 66. The opacification of the right hemithorax soon after insertion of a central line should make you question whether the line ends in the pleural space rather than in the superior vena cava or right atrium. In other words, is the opacification caused by a massive accumulation of TPN fluid in the pleural space? In fact, there is so much fluid present that the right lung is compressed and the mediastinum is shifted to the left.

The position of the central venous line could have been determined by contrast injection through the line the previous day, and, indeed, this is routinely performed in some institutions. In this case, close inspection of the initial radiograph obtained soon after TPN administration showed fluid in the horizontal fissure. This fluid accumulation required an explanation, and a radiograph with "overpenetrated technique" and contrast injection would have given an immediate answer!

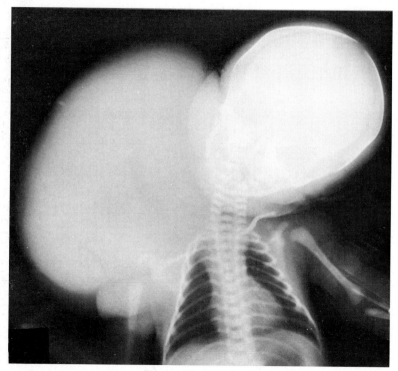

Baby Boy Amadeus was born by cesarean section because of dystocia resulting from a neck mass. Any thoughts as to the nature of this mass?

Figure 67. Amadeus

ANSWER

The radiograph shows a huge homogeneous soft tissue mass arising from *Baby Amadeus'* neck. Neither fat nor calcification is present in the mass, and physical examination showed it to arise from the posterior triangle of the neck. The mass was firm and lobulated and permitted transillumination.

This is the classic appearance and location of a congenital malformation of the lymph channels known as cystic hygroma. This lesion may involve the mediastinum and the axilla and requires resection to prevent compression of adjacent structures and possible infection.

A condition to be considered in the differential diagnosis of a lateral neck mass is the branchial cleft cyst. A midline neck mass should make you think of an enlargement of the thyroid gland or of a thyroglossal duct cyst.

IS HIS HEART IN THE RIGHT PLACE?

Jay M., 1 month old, has an abnormal appearance in that he has a small head with eyes that appear to slant upward and outward, eyelids with thick epicanthal folds, a thickened tongue, separation of the first and second toes, and a single deep transverse crease across the palm; he also has a heart murmur. Also, his heart sounds are heard better in the right hemithorax.

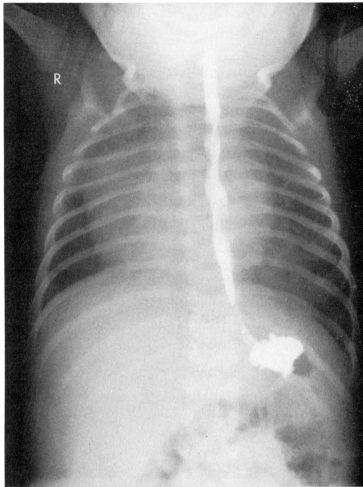

Figure 68. Jay M.

Figure 69. David S.

David S. is a 1 month old boy who was examined at a well baby clinic, where he appeared to be completely healthy (except for a mild diaper rash). However, the pediatrician had felt a mass in the left upper quadrant of the abdomen.

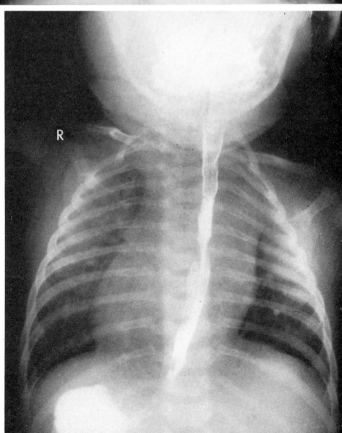

ANSWERS

David S. and *Jay M.* both have dextrocardia. This means that the cardiac apex points to the right (the main muscle mass of the heart is to the right of the spine).

In *David S.'* case, there is also situs inversus of the abdominal viscera, meaning that the patient's stomach is on his right side and the liver is on the left side (the "mass" felt by the pediatrician was, of course, the liver).

Jay M., on the other hand, has his liver on the right side and the stomach on the left side, where they ought to be. This is termed situs solitus, the position of the abdominal organs being normal.

The term applied to *David S.'* condition is mirror-image dextrocardia. Additional cardiac malformations are rarely encountered. No such abnormality was found in *David,* whose growth and development have been unremarkable.

Jay M. has "situs solitus with dextrocardia." This situation is usually associated with complex congenital heart disease, and it is rarely possible to make a precise anatomic diagnosis without cardiac catheterization. *Jay,* in fact, has Down's syndrome, or trisomy 21. This condition is often associated with an "endocardial cushion defect." This term refers to the four centers of growth from which parts of the mitral and tricuspid valves as well as the contiguous portions of the atrial and ventricular septa are formed. A defect in the endocardial cushions leads to a left-to-right shunt.

Although *Jay* has an endocardial cushion defect, it is more common for patients with situs solitus and dextrocardia to have "corrected transposition of the great vessels," ventricular septal defect with pulmonary stenosis, tricuspid atresia, or other malformations. In other words, usually you can't predict the congenital heart disease in patients with situs solitus and dextrocardia.

When you consider the diagnosis of Down's syndrome or trisomy 21, scrutinize the sternum on the lateral chest radiograph (Figs. 70 and 71). A double ossification center of the manubrium is seen in a high percentage of such patients. However, since this finding can also be seen in normal children, you must be cautious in how you use this information.

Figure 70.

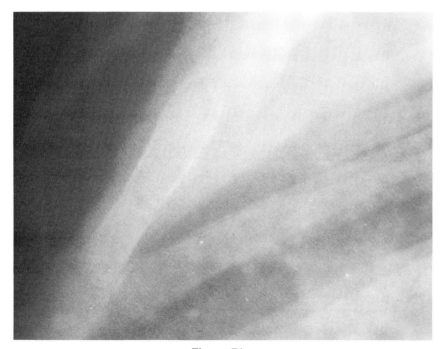

Figure 71.

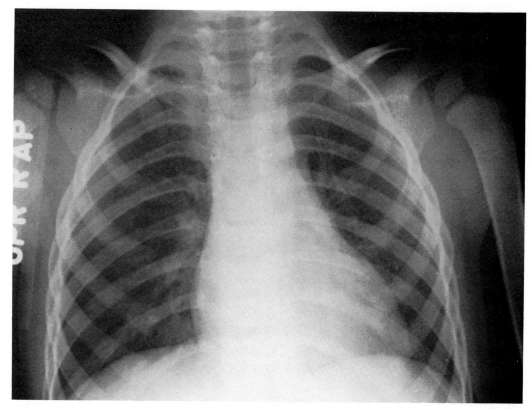

Figure 72. Michael B.

Michael B. is a 2 year old boy who appeared to his parents to be in perfect health. However, during a routine physical examination his pediatrician found the blood pressure in the arms to be 140/90 mm Hg, while the blood pressure in the legs was unobtainable. The femoral pulses were present but diminished.

The examination of the chest revealed that the point of maximal impulse was in the fourth intercostal space at the midclavicular line. A grade ii/iv midsystolic murmur was heard.

The AP chest radiograph is presented here (Fig. 72).

ANSWER

Michael's physicians agreed that clinically he had a coarctation of the aorta. They consulted with the surgeons and radiologists and felt that aortography was indicated to define the extent and site of the coarctation. Figure 73 is one "cut" from the aortogram. The catheter can be seen entering the aortic arch from the right subclavian artery.

There is a localized constriction in the descending thoracic aorta inferior to the site at which the ductus would be seen if it were patent and opacified. This is termed "adult" or post-ductal coarctation, as opposed to pre-ductal or "infantile" coarctation. In post-ductal coarctation there is a 75 per cent incidence of bicuspid aortic valve, which *Michael* had. (This is significant because of the incidence of subacute bacterial endocarditis in bicuspid aortic valves.)

Examination of the extensive collateral circulation in this coarctation of the aorta reveals strikingly dilated and tortuous vessels, including the internal mammary arteries and the thyrocervical trunks. Fortunately, there is communication between the collateral circulation above the level of the coarctation and that which is below the coarctation, thereby ensuring an adequate supply of blood to the lower part of the body despite the reduced blood flow in the aorta.

Why did *Michael* have hypertension? One theory is that the constriction of the aorta causes hypertension on a renal basis, rather like a Goldblatt kidney preparation. Another hypothesis suggests that the hypertension is caused by mechanical factors. There is increased resistance and reduced distensibility of the aorta above the constriction, which may well explain the hypertension in the arms. Actually, both factors may be significant.

The plain films of the chest usually show only mild cardiomegaly. Rib notching, caused by erosion of the ribs resulting from the enlarged intercostal arteries, is rarely seen under the age of 5 and is barely detectable here. Occasionally

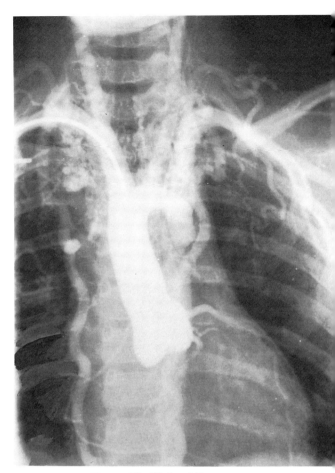

Figure 73. Michael B.

the ascending aorta may be prominent, and if a barium swallow is done, there may be a projection on the contour of the barium-opacified esophagus at the site of the coarctation.

When *Michael* was 7 years old, he was operated upon and the coarcted segment was removed. An end-to-end anastomosis of the remaining thoracic aorta was performed. The reason that the child was not operated upon at the time of diagnosis was that there was some concern that the region of the anastomosis might not grow. It is preferable to wait until the child and aorta are bigger. Of course, if the child shows early evidence of congestive heart failure, the procedure may be performed when he is younger.

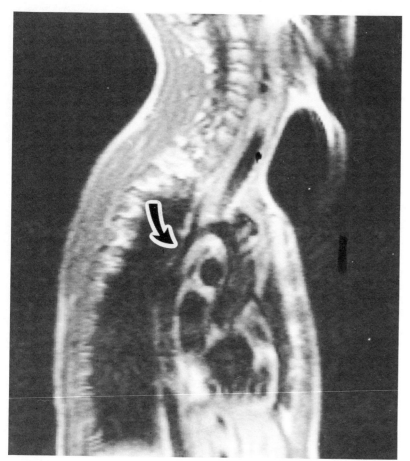

Figure 74.

The patient in Figure 74 also has coarctation of the aorta. The arrow indicates the narrowing of the proximal descending aorta, demonstrated on this magnetic resonance image (MRI). Vessels are clearly seen by MRI, since no signal is produced by moving blood.

A SEVEN YEAR OLD WITH CYANOSIS

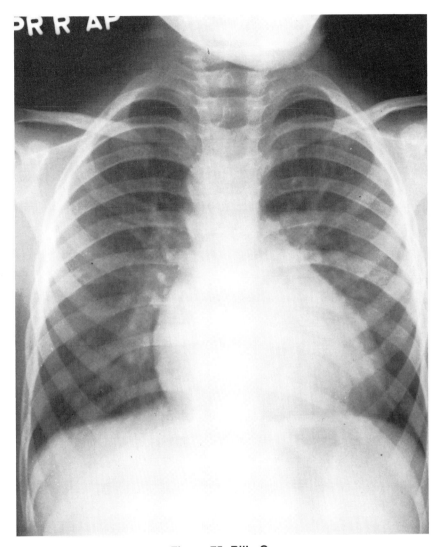

Figure 75. Billy G.

Billy G., now 7 years old, was noted at birth to have a cardiac murmur associated with slight but definite cyanosis. At that time he was admitted to another hospital, where a diagnosis of congenital heart disease was made. Treatment with digitalis was begun and was continued until age 4. Since then, *Billy* has done well, with minimal cyanosis and normal growth and development. Recently, however, he has begun to have decreased exercise tolerance and increasing cyanosis. He is now admitted for cardiac catheterization and consideration for surgical correction (Fig. 75).

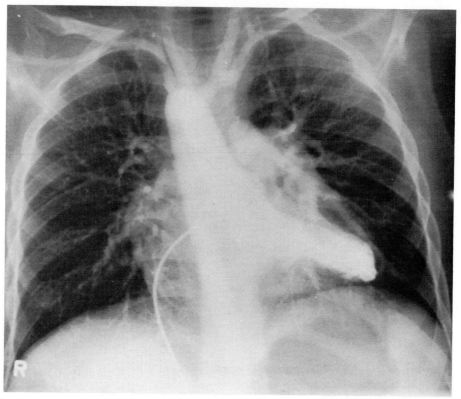

Figure 76. Billy G.

ANSWER

The chest radiograph on *Billy* showed normal arrangement of the abdominal viscera. This is implied by the position of the stomach bubble on the patient's left.

Which side is the aortic arch on? Look carefully at the tracheal air shadow. It is deviated slightly to the left. This tells you that the aortic arch is on the right side, and indeed, you can see a rounded density projected over the right fourth interspace. Also, there is no room for the normal aortic arch to the left of the trachea.

The pulmonary vascularity is about normal. The heart size and shape are also normal.

In summary, the plain AP chest radiograph shows normal abdominal situs, normal size and shape of the heart, normal pulmonary vascularity, and a right-sided aortic arch. Figure 76 is one frame of an angiogram that confirms the presence of the right aortic arch. How was the injection made? Are there more findings on the angiogram? What's the diagnosis?

ANSWER (*Continued*)

The analysis of any angiogram begins with the position of the catheter, which is seen in Figure 77 with a radiopaque marker on its tip. The lateral view (Fig. 78) shows the right ventricle positioned anteriorly, receiving the injection of contrast material.

The infundibulum is the part of the right ventricular outflow tract just superior to the catheter tip. The tight stenosis seen in both the AP and lateral views is characteristic of this form of congenital heart disease. Sometimes pulmonary valvar stenosis occurs in addition to the infundibular stenosis (and, rarely, there may be total absence of the pulmonary valve).

Figure 76 shows simultaneous opacification of the aorta and pulmonary artery, which occurs because of a ventricular septal defect that permits contrast material and blood to flow from the right ventricle to the left ventricle. In Figure 76 you can barely see the infundibular stenosis.

Billy has tetralogy of Fallot. About one fourth of these patients will have a right-sided aortic arch. Other features of this condition include stenosis of the right ventricular outflow tract, usually at the infundibular level but sometimes at the valvar level or at both levels. This results in right ventricular hypertrophy. There is also a ventricular septal defect, and the aorta overrides both ventricular cavities.

Infants with tetralogy of Fallot are usually initially treated medically until they are older and bigger and are better able to tolerate surgery. Small, frequent feedings and oxygen and morphine for the "blue spells" are important. Nonetheless, some infants will have "blue spells" so often that surgery is mandatory. Direct anastomosis of the aorta to the pulmonary artery will supply more blood to the lungs and can be performed in infancy. The Blalock-Taussig operation is another shunt procedure in which the subclavian artery is anastomosed to

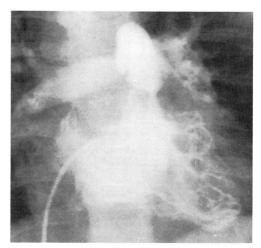

Figure 77. Billy G.

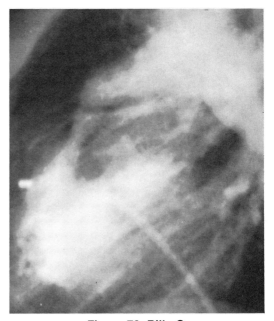

Figure 78. Billy G.

the main branch of the pulmonary artery.

Billy had a "total correction" procedure. This consists of closure of the ventricular septal defect, resection of the infundibular stenosis (or enlargement of the volume of the infundibulum with a pericardial patch), and relief of any pulmonic valvar stenosis via valvulotomy. *Billy* has done well clinically since surgery and is now an active child who is gaining weight and growing normally.

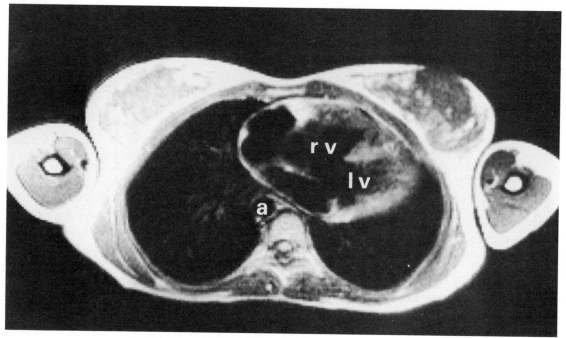

Figure 79.

This MRI study on another youngster (Fig. 79) with tetralogy of Fallot shows a right-sided descending aorta (a) and a large ventricular septal defect (VSD). (lv = left ventricle; rv = right ventricle.)

Another axial MRI study (Fig. 80) at a slightly higher level demonstrates a large overriding aortic root (aa) and hypoplastic pulmonary arteries (arrows).

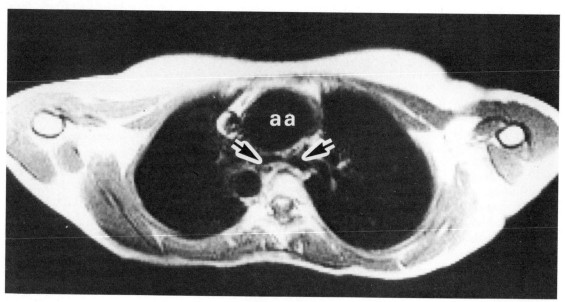

Figure 80.

A TWO YEAR OLD WITH CYANOSIS

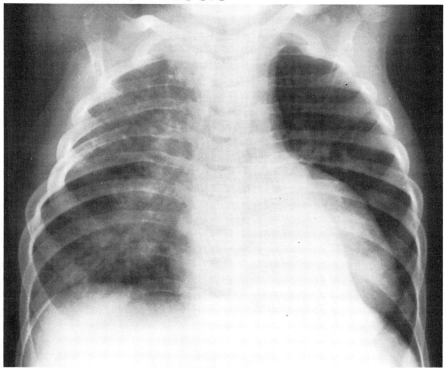

Figure 81. Philip G.

Philip G. is a 2 year old boy with cough, fever, and cyanosis who is brought to the Emergency Room by the baby sitter because of his obviously ill appearance. The parents are on vacation, but the baby sitter thinks the child has been seen before at this hospital. A chest x-ray is requested while the record room looks for the old chart.

The x-ray requisition states, "R/O pneumonia." (Further clinical data would have been a help!) How would you report this chest AP and lateral (Figs. 81 and 82)?

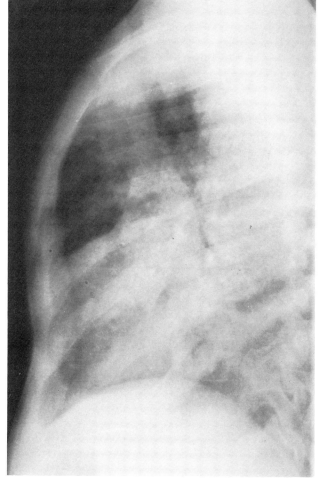

Figure 82. Philip G.

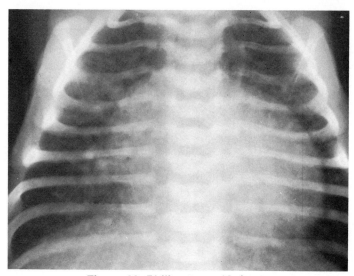

Figure 83. Philip at age 13 days

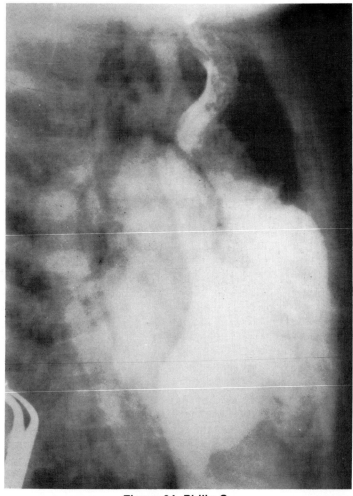

Figure 84. Philip G.

ANSWER

Philip clearly has a triangular-shaped density superimposed on the left cardiac silhouette; this density represents a collapsed left lower lobe.

The heart appears enlarged, and the right fourth and fifth ribs look different from the other ribs. A rib that appears different from its brothers may simply be reflecting the footprints of the cardiac surgeon. Certainly, a large heart and rib changes would be consistent with some form of surgically treated congenital heart disease, and usually old films prior to surgery are helpful in establishing the radiologic diagnosis. In *Philip's* case, the file room came up with the master folder; Figure 83 shows *Philip* at age 13 days.

The base of the heart ("vascular pedicle") is very narrow, and the pulmonary vascularity is definitely increased. The triad of a cyanotic patient whose chest radiograph shows increased vascularity and a narrow vascular pedicle should suggest the diagnosis, which is confirmed on the lateral view of the venous angiogram (Fig. 84). Contrast material is seen in the superior vena cava entering the heart, but note that the aorta is anterior to the pulmonary artery. In case you don't recall, this is abnormal; the normal situation consists of the pulmonary artery anterior to the aorta as seen on the lateral view. Because the great arteries are reversed in location, it can be stated that *Philip* has transposition of the great arteries. The aorta arises from the right ventricle, and the pulmonary artery arises from the left ventricle. This situation is not compatible with life (think about it!) unless there is mixing of the blood via a shunt such as an atrial septal defect, ventricular septal defect, or patent ductus arteriosus.

Philip had a ventricular septal defect, but to increase the mixing a Rashkind procedure was performed during the first weeks of his life. This procedure consists of enlarging the patent foramen ovale by pulling a balloon-tipped catheter back through it during cardiac catheterization. This is a temporary measure intended to create enough mixing of blood so that the child can survive until he is old enough for corrective surgery.

The rib change is indeed evidence that open heart surgery was performed, in this case a Blalock-Hanlen procedure. This is the creation of a permanent interatrial communication intended to further improve mixing of blood. (This information was gained by reading the x-ray reports from the film master file. Sometimes if the patient's chart is missing, you can learn a great deal about the patient's prior history from the x-ray reports in the master file.)

At this point we know that *Philip* has transposition of the great vessels that was treated with a Rashkind procedure and with a Blalock-Hanlen operation. He has "overcirculation" in the pulmonary circuit (remember the increase in pulmonary vascularity), resulting in an increase in the size of the left atrium. When the left atrium is exceedingly enlarged in infants, it compresses the left lower lobe bronchus, causing atelectasis. (Other radiologists think that the collapse is due to the enlarged heart.) Obviously, this is difficult to treat, and a series of old films all showed a loss of volume of the left lower lobe to a greater or lesser degree.

Why is the "vascular pedicle" narrowed in Figure 83? With transposition of the great arteries, the ascending aorta is displaced, so that in the frontal projection it superposes the descending aorta. Moreover, the thymus is atrophic. By the way, did you notice that the aorta is narrowed distal to the branching of the great vessels (Fig. 84)? If not, you missed a coarctation of the aorta.

Figure 85 is an axial MRI study at the great vessel level in a child with transposition of the great arteries. The ascending aorta (A) is anterior to the pulmonary artery (PA), the reverse of normal.

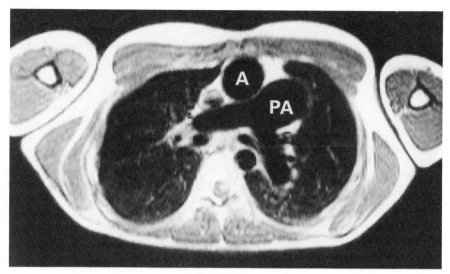

Figure 85.

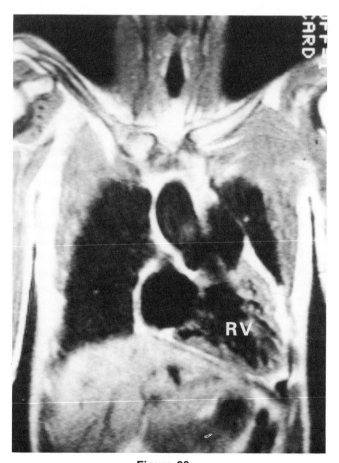

Figure 86.

A coronal MRI study in the same patient is illustrated in Figure 86. Note that the aortic root arises from the thick-walled, trabeculated right ventricle (RV). You *do* remember that this is abnormal, don't you?

Abdomen

THREE PATIENTS WITH FEVER AND ABDOMINAL PAIN...

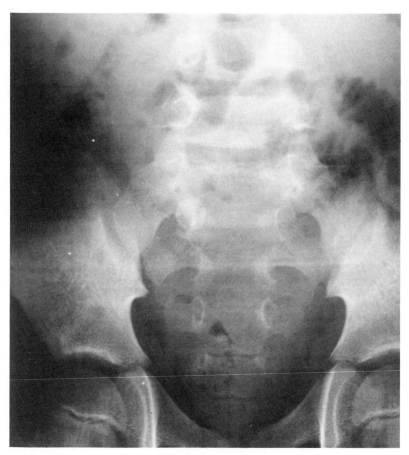

Figure 87. T. Hope

Trelawney Hope, age 12, the great grandson of the Right Honorable Trelawney Hope, was visiting the United States with his rock group called the "Stones" (he plays the electric harmonica) when he became ill. Initially he developed vague abdominal pain and nausea, which he attributed to a change in diet. After several hours he began to vomit, and the pain migrated to the right lower quadrant of the abdomen. The manager of the rock group took the boy to the emergency room of the nearest hospital.

Physical examination confirmed tenderness in the right lower quadrant of the abdomen. A rectal examination suggested a mass in the same region.

Temperature, 99.8° F (orally); pulse, 100 beats per minute; respiration, 16 breaths per minute; WBC 9000— normal differential.

Mlle. H. Fournaye, age 11, also a member of the "Stones," had exactly the same symptoms as *Trelawney Hope*. She had no abdominal tenderness and definitely no signs of peritoneal irritation. The only positive physical findings were reduced hearing (probably nerve deafness, an occupational hazard) and dullness on percussion with bronchial breath sounds in the right lower lobe area.

Temperature, 103° F (orally); pulse, 120 beats per minute; respiration, 28 breaths per minute; WBC 28,000.

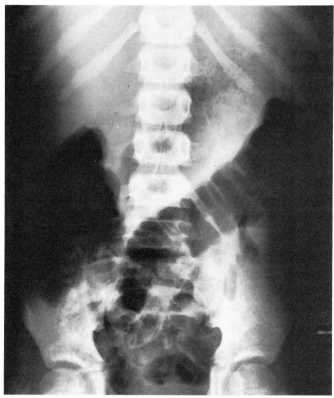

Figure 88. Mlle. H. Fournaye

Eduardo Lucas, of West Indian descent and also a member of the English rock group the "Stones," had a urinary tract infection. Figure 89 was the preliminary radiograph for an intravenous pyelogram (IVP).

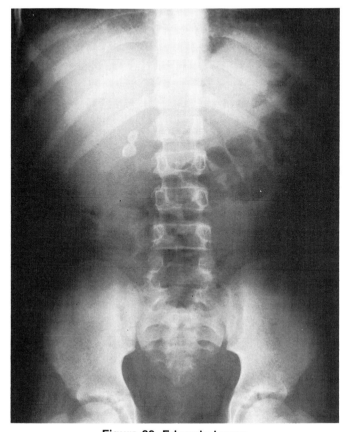

Figure 89. Eduardo Lucas

ANSWERS

Look carefully at the right lower quadrant of *Trelawney Hope's* radiograph, and you will see a calcific density superimposed on the sacrum. This shadow represents a fecalith, indicates appendicitis, and requires surgery.

Other radiologic findings of appendicitis (not seen here) include ileus of the terminal ileum and a soft tissue fullness in the right lower quadrant, indicative of a mass. (This is seen especially in patients with periappendiceal abscess.)

At surgery there was a pinpoint perforation in the tip of the appendix, around which there was a small abscess containing the fecalith. Recovery was slow because of the perforation, but now *Trelawney* is again blowing the electric harmonica with his rock group. He has subsequently changed the name of his group from the "Stones" to the "Appendicoliths."

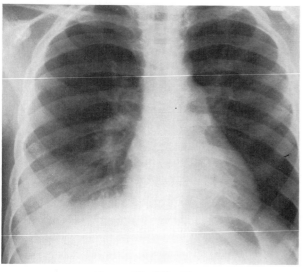

Figure 90. Mlle. Fournaye

Mlle. Fournaye's supine view of the abdomen is normal. (Yes, we worried that there might be fecaliths in the right lower quadrant, but a coned-down view of that area showed only small fecal masses and gas in the cecum and ascending colon.)

A patient with abdominal pain requires chest radiographs because lower lobe pneumonia may cause diaphragmatic irritation and referral of pain to the abdomen. Figure 90 shows just that: consolidation in the right lower lobe.

After Gram stain of the sputum and cultures, *Mlle. Fournaye* was started on antibiotic therapy. Her fever remitted promptly, and she still possesses her appendix. Unfortunately, her hearing continues to deteriorate, but she is proud of this because she feels a common bond with Beethoven.

Eduardo was known to have sickle cell anemia, and one of the manifestations of this disease is gallstone formation. Figure 89 shows two faceted gallstones in the right upper quadrant of the abdomen. Other anemias, including thalassemia and acquired hemolytic anemias, may also be complicated by gallstone formation.

Some of the other manifestations of sickle cell disease include formation of thrombi in various organs, cardiomegaly, and infarction of bone, brain, lungs, kidney, or spleen. These children are particularly susceptible to *Salmonella* infection.

In the case of *Eduardo*, the gallstones were an incidental finding on the preliminary film of the IVP, which showed clearly that the stones were not in the kidney. Presence of the stones in the gallbladder was proved by ultrasonography. He had no symptoms of cholelithiasis, and he has not yet had a cholecystectomy. His fever and abdominal pain were secondary to his urinary tract infection.

... AND TWO MORE CHILDREN WITH ABDOMINAL PAIN

Percy Trevelyan, a 3 year old boy, was feeling completely well, according to his mother, when he suddenly developed abdominal pain. The boy subsequently passed a bloody stool, which alarmed Mrs. Trevelyan and caused her to bring the boy to the hospital.

The physical examination revealed an acutely ill child in obvious pain but with normal vital signs. There was a mass in the right lower quadrant of the abdomen that was soft and only minimally tender. There was no rigidity or rebound tenderness. Otherwise, the abdominal examination was negative. The pediatrician put the clinical history together with the physical findings and made a tentative diagnosis. He sent the boy to the Radiology Department for confirmation *and* treatment.

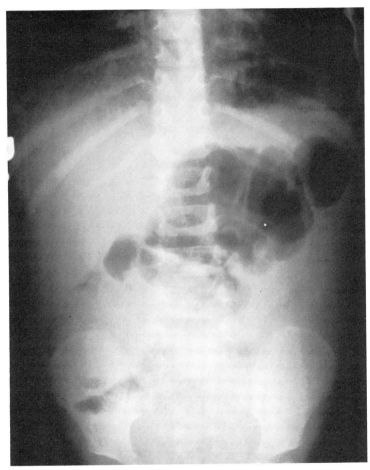

Figure 91. Percy Trevelyan

A 13 year old girl, **Miss Blessington,** appeared one afternoon in the Emergency Room complaining of urgency and frequency of urination accompanied by pain in the suprapubic region. She had been seen in the Child Psychiatry Clinic because of a behavior disorder, and the intern wondered if her symptoms weren't simply a part of her pattern of behavior.

The physical examination was negative, but a urinalysis showed WBCs and bacteria TNTC (too numerous to count). An IVP was requested, and Figure 92 is part of the preliminary plain film of the abdomen. After seeing this film, the intern requested a urologic consultation, suspecting that this child had bladder stones. The radiologist questioned the child and took another radiograph, which confirmed the diagnosis. What question did he ask *Miss Blessington,* and what radiograph did he obtain?

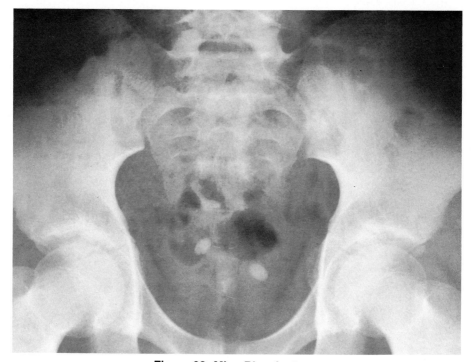

Figure 92. Miss Blessington

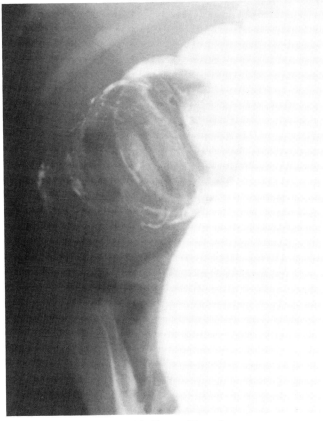

Figure 93. Percy Trevelyan

ANSWERS

Percy's radiologic workup was begun with a supine view of the abdomen (Fig. 91). This showed a soft tissue density in the right lower quadrant of the abdomen consistent with an ileocolic intussusception. In this condition, the proximal bowel telescopes into the distal bowel. It may sometimes be caused by a polyp or Meckel's diverticulum, but often no cause is found for the intussusception.

Initial treatment consists of confirmation of the diagnosis and hydrostatic reduction of the intussusception by means of barium enema. Care is taken to ensure that no pressure is exerted on the abdomen or the barium bag, and that the enema tube is not "milked." The barium bag is adjusted to a height of 2½ feet above the x-ray table. A "spot film" (Fig. 93) shows the "coiled spring" appearance that is characteristic of intussusception.

Reduction is considered to be complete when there is free flow of barium into the small bowel from a normally filled cecum. If this can't be demonstrated, surgical reduction will be necessary; however, in about two thirds to three fourths of the cases of intussusception, the barium enema will be both diagnostic *and* therapeutic.

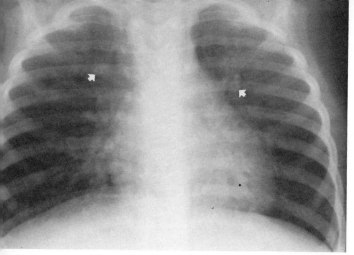

Figure 94. Percy Trevelyan

Percy also has cystic fibrosis, which you can recognize from the chest film (Fig. 94) and from the edge of the abdominal film (Fig. 91) because of the peribronchial cuffing seen well overlying the right fourth rib posteriorly and left fifth rib posteriorly. Changes are also visible in the lung bases, as shown in Figure 91. Cystic fibrosis is a known, but not common, cause of intussusception. In *Percy's* case, the intussusception could not be reduced with a barium enema, and surgery was necessary.

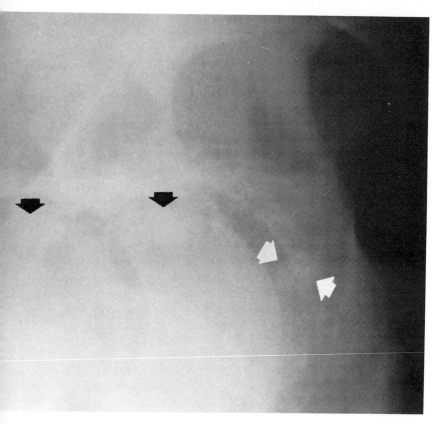

Figure 95. Miss Blessington

Bladder stones are uncommon in children in the absence of a neurogenic bladder or severe chronic infection. The radiologist obtained a lateral view of *Miss Blessington* (Fig. 95), which showed the densities to be posterior and in the rectum (white arrows). The black arrows indicate the not-quite-superimposed femoral heads. He then questioned *Miss Blessington* and learned that she had been receiving iron tablets for the treatment of excessive menstrual bleeding. She showed him the tablets, and they corresponded in size and shape to the densities seen in Figure 92.

It turned out that the child also had cystitis, and this accounted for her symptoms and urinalysis findings. An IVP was not performed.

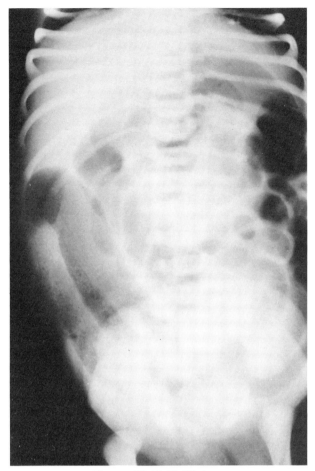

Figure 96. B. B. Watson

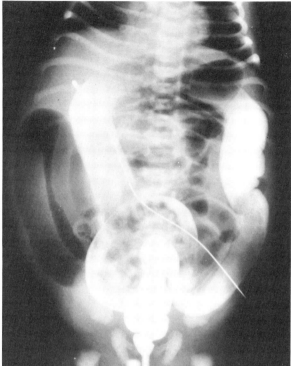

Figure 97. B. B. Watson

Baby Boy Watson is a 2 day old infant who has not yet passed a meconium stool. Because the plain radiograph of the abdomen showed multiple dilated bowel loops, intestinal obstruction was suspected and an enema using water-soluble contrast material was performed. What does it show? Are those filling defects in the colon normal?

ANSWER

The pertinent findings are the large filling defects within the colon, which represent ribbons of meconium. It is said that such plugs are present in about 1 per cent of all newborns. Seventy-five per cent of the time, they are passed spontaneously. In those infants in whom the plugs are retained, the water-soluble contrast enema is therapeutic. Because of the high osmolality of the enema content, fluid is pulled into the colonic lu-men, facilitating passage of the meconium.

It is very important to know that 5 per cent of infants with the so-called meconium plug syndrome at birth have Hirschsprung's disease. Thus, these babies should be watched carefully for the development of constipation. In addition, there is a higher-than-normal incidence of cystic fibrosis in infants with the meconium plug syndrome.

TWO BABIES WITH VOMITING AND DEHYDRATION

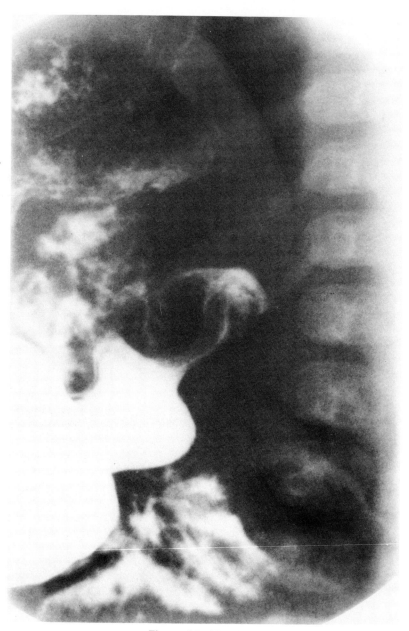

Figure 98. Alec C.

Alec Cunningham, 3 weeks old, developed projectile vomiting (this means that the vomitus clears the chin and distinguishes it from drooling) during the second week of life. His abdomen became distended, and peristaltic waves were clearly visible through the abdominal wall.

When first seen at the hospital, this boy was dehydrated. Examination of the abdomen suggested a tumor mass, the size of an olive, in the region of the outlet of the stomach.

The surgical resident was sufficiently uncertain of the diagnosis to request an upper gastrointestinal series to confirm his impression (Fig. 98).

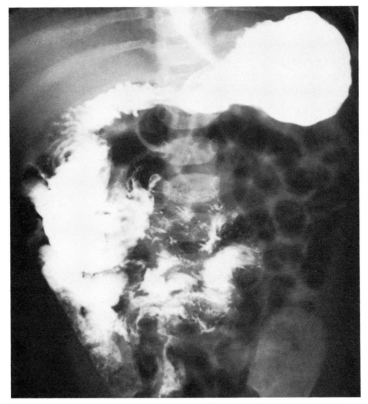

Figure 99. Baron Maupertuis

Baron Maupertuis, a 7 month old boy, was brought to his pediatrician because of bile-stained vomitus. He had had intermittent abdominal pains and vomiting before, and now his mother was alarmed by the return of his symptoms.

The *Baron* appeared ill and weighed only 9 lb. 14 oz. (an increase of only 2 lb. 14 oz. since birth). His vital signs were normal, but the child was mildly dehydrated. His abdomen was tender, but there were no signs of peritoneal irritation.

The *Baron* was admitted to the hospital, and an upper gastrointestinal series was performed (Fig. 99).

ANSWERS

The striking feature of *Alec Cunningham's* upper gastrointestinal series is the extreme length of the pyloric channel. The ribbon-like strips of barium extending from the antrum to the duodenal bulb are explained by the fact that the pyloric canal is not a circular tube; instead, the mucosa has many longitudinal folds in which the barium is trapped. When radiographed, as in Figure 98, the barium in the canal therefore has a ribbon-like or railroad track appearance.

This, then, is hypertrophic pyloric stenosis. It is much more common in males than in females and usually develops several weeks after birth. In this condition the circular pyloric muscle is hypertrophied, with secondary narrowing of the pyloric canal and redundancy of the mucosa.

The etiology is unknown, but there is a distinct familial tendency. The diagnosis is established upon palpation of the "pyloric olive." Only rarely, perhaps in 1 case in 10, will an upper gastrointestinal series be necessary, and only then because the history is confusing or the physical examination equivocal. In some centers, ultrasonographic evaluation has replaced the barium study as the first imaging modality in infants with suspected pyloric stenosis.

In the past, medical management (antispasmodics and thickened feedings) was used to treat hypertrophic pyloric stenosis. Today, the Ramstedt pyloromyotomy is the treatment of choice. In this operation a lengthwise incision is made through the hypertrophied pyloric muscle, and the mucosa is allowed to prolapse through the incised area. This relieves the gastric outlet obstruction, and almost invariably the symptoms promptly disappear.

The *Baron's* upper gastrointestinal series and the coned-down view of the duodenum show an abnormal position of the third and fourth portions of the duodenum and of the duodenal-jejunal junction. The third portion should pass horizontally from the right to the left of the spine, and the fourth portion should ascend so that the duodenal-jejunal junction is at the same height as the junction of the first and second portions of the duodenum. In the *Baron*, the duodenal-jejunal junction is displaced downward and to the right of the spine. The malposition of the distal one half of the duodenum is the tip-off that the Baron has intestinal malrotation.

The fetal gastrointestinal tract is a straight tube initially. At the fifth week of fetal life the midgut (which comprises the distal duodenum, the small bowel, and about the proximal one half of the colon) elongates and soon herniates into what will become the umbilical cord. At the same time, the cecum moves to the patient's left and the duodenum-jejunum to the patient's right, as rotation of the midgut begins. The duodenum and the colon are close together at this point. If rotation arrests at this stage of development, or at any subsequent stage before the duodenal-jejunal junction is in the normal location, bands frequently form between the duodenum and colon. Also, the attachment of the small bowel mesentery about the origin of the superior mesenteric artery is abnormal and predisposes to midgut volvulus with the superior mesenteric artery as the axis for the twist.

Figure 100 shows a barium enema performed in an infant with early arrest in the process of intestinal rotation. As you can see, the cecum is located in the left upper quadrant. Figure 101 is an upper gastrointestinal series performed on another infant who has duodenal obstruction (arrow) resulting from "Ladd's bands."

The *Baron* has one of the two complications of malrotation. The bands, frequently referred to as Ladd's bands, extend from the right colon across the duodenum to the upper abdomen and cause intermittent extrinsic compression of the duodenum, obstruction, and bilious vomiting.

The second complication of malrotation is volvulus of the midgut about the superior mesenteric artery. This is allowed by the incomplete fixation of the small bowel mesentery and may result

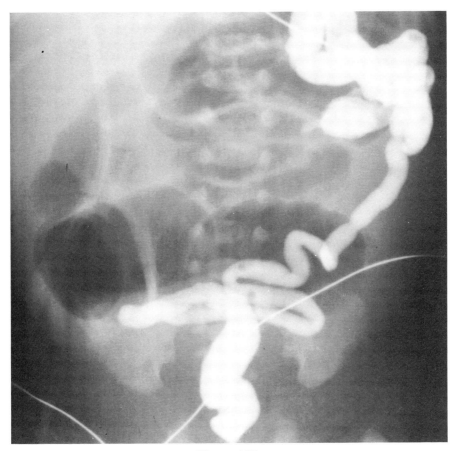

Figure 100.

in infarction of the midgut. A third and rarer complication is chronic malabsorption.

About one half of the patients with malrotation are seen in the first week of life. The remaining cases are present throughout childhood and sometimes into adulthood.

The *Baron* had surgical correction of the malrotation. The "Ladd's bands" compressing the duodenum were divided. The intestine was inspected; volvulus had not developed. Then the intestines were returned to the abdominal cavity and the ascending colon was fixed on the left side and the duodenum-jejunum was fixed on the right side. This position has been found to prevent volvulus later on.

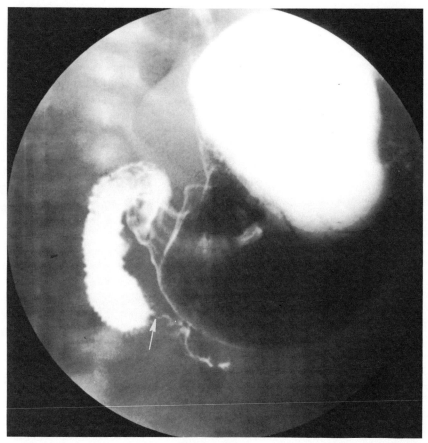

Figure 101.

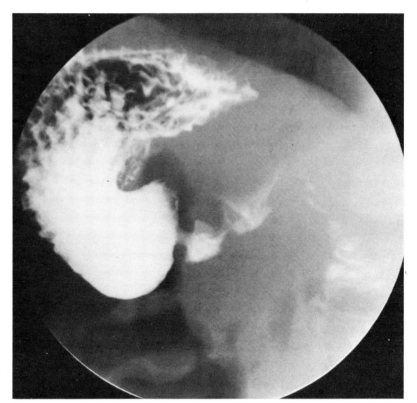

Sherlock H. is a 4 year old boy with a long history of vomiting and failure to thrive. His spot radiograph taken during an upper gastrointestinal series solves the mystery of Sherlock's illness.

Figure 102. Sherlock H.

ANSWER

Did you locate one or two successive pyloric canals? Well, there seems to be two, don't you agree? The distal one is the real pyloric canal; the proximal constricted column of barium represents a stream of barium as it goes through a central perforation in an antral web. This relatively uncommon congenital anomaly consists of a circumferential mucosal membrane with a variable-sized opening. The degree of obstruction produced is also variable, and patients with this abnormality may be symptomatic for a relatively long time before a diagnosis is made. If the symptoms warrant, surgery is performed to relieve gastric outlet obstruction. *However*, endoscopy should be done first, as false-positive "pseudowebs" are occasionally mistaken for the real thing on the upper gastrointestinal series!

TWO CHILDREN WITH ABDOMINAL CRAMPS AND DIARRHEA

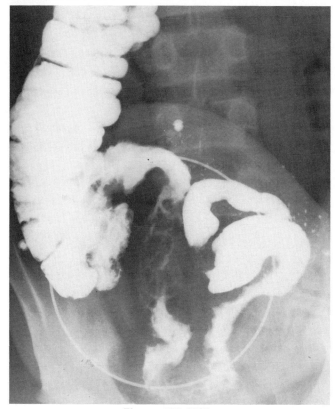

Figure 103. Willy

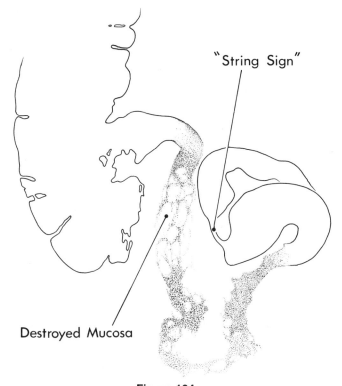

Figure 104.

Willy (full name: **Wilhelm Gottsreich Sigismond von Ormstein,** Grand Duke of Cassel-Falstein and hereditary King of Bohemia), age 14, had a history of several years of cramping abdominal pain associated with fever and diarrhea. The diarrhea was accompanied by excessive mucus in the stools and, rarely, blood. His weight gain had been slow, and he appeared chronically ill.

Physical examination revealed a small boy, slender and somewhat cachectic. The oral temperature was 99.6° F, but the other vital signs were normal. The pertinent physical findings included tenderness in the right lower quadrant, where there was an ill-defined mass. There were no rectal fistulas. A barium enema was performed, at which time reflux occurred into the terminal ileum (Fig. 103).

Clotilde Lothman (full name; von Saxe-Meningen, second daughter of the king of Scandinavia), age 16, was incapacitated by bloody diarrhea occurring about 15 times daily. The feces were watery and contained pus and mucus as well as blood. The diarrhea was accompanied by cramping abdominal pain.

Physical examination showed a chronically ill child. She had had iritis and arthritis in the past.

Her abdomen was diffusely tender, but no mass could be palpated. There was also no evidence of peritoneal irritation or of cutaneous fistulas. The radiographs presented here are the AP and left anterior oblique views of the abdomen obtained during barium enema examination (Figs. 105 and 106).

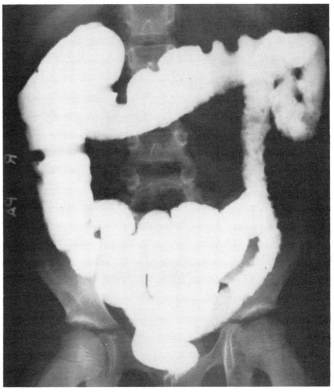

Figure 105. Clotilde Lothman

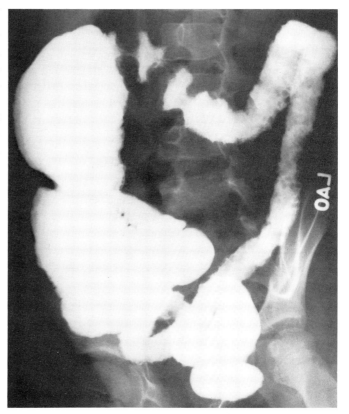

Figure 106. Clotilde Lothman

ANSWERS

The radiologist doing *Willy's* barium enema has used a pressure paddle with a metallic rim to separate the loops of terminal ileum. In the center of the field encompassed by the pressure paddle there is an area of ileum in which the intestinal lumen shows irregular coating with barium and destruction of the normal mucosal pattern. The more proximal ileum appears normal except for a short involved area. The "skipping" of areas of involvement is typical of this condition, as is the markedly narrowed lumen, seen best in the proximal area of involvement. Because the lumen is no wider than string, this has been termed the "string sign."

At fluoroscopy, the radiologist looked for fistulas and for involvement of the cecum. The right lower quadrant of the abdomen was quite tender during palpation with the pressure paddle, but colonic involvement and fistulas were not found.

Willy has regional enteritis (Crohn's disease). This condition characteristically involves discrete segments of the small bowel. Initially the bowel wall is thickened, and becomes stenosed and fibrotic in the late stages of the disease. The process is accompanied by apparent obstruction of the lymphatics and thickening of the mesentery. Microscopically, noncaseating granulomas are seen deep in the bowel wall. Areas of necrosis may occur, and fistulas may form.

The etiology of regional enteritis is unknown. The classic clinical presentation of diarrhea and cramps is not always seen, especially in children. Some children present with growth failure and are found to have a delayed bone age, so that hypopituitarism is suspected. Other children are seen because of rectal fistulas or intestinal obstruction, while still others have symptoms that suggest acute appendicitis. The stomach, duodenum, jejunum, and colon as well as the ileum may be involved, and the symptoms will vary accordingly.

Treatment consists of a low-residue diet and a nonabsorbable sulfonamide, salicylazosulfapyridine (Azulfidine). Steroids have occasionally been used. Surgery is ordinarily reserved for controlling the complications of regional enteritis, such as bowel obstruction, fistulas, and perforation.

Willy continues to exist in symbiosis with his disease, which he regards as a chronic disability. He and his physicians do not think in terms of cure but in terms of long-term control of the symptoms. At the time this is written, the child is able to participate in school, but his grades suffer from frequent absences. His parents are concerned that progression of the disease will eventually restrict his activities and limit his ability to attend school and participate in normal childhood activities.

Clotilde was admitted to the hospital. A barium enema was performed only after preliminary views of the abdomen showed no evidence of "toxic megacolon." (The clinical diagnosis was ulcerative colitis, and if the bowel had become acutely dilated and friable, this condition would have been termed toxic megacolon. In this situation, a barium enema might perforate the colon and spill barium into the peritoneal cavity.) The AP, left anterior oblique, and coned-down views (Fig. 107) of the descending colon show deep and superficial ulcers in the bowel wall. The diameter of the lumen of the descending colon is reduced, and no haustrations are seen.

Clotilde has not only the clinical but also the radiologic findings of ulcerative colitis. The disease ordinarily begins in the rectum or sigmoid colon, which are better evaluated by proctoscopy and sigmoidoscopy than by barium enema.

The mucosa can be inspected through the proctoscope or sigmoidoscope and will be found to bleed easily. Minute ulcers in the mucosa may be detected as well. Later the ulcers may coalesce, so that the islands of remaining mucosa appear as pseudopolyps. As the disease progresses, the bowel becomes shortened, with "lead pipe rigidity." In children with a history of ulcerative colitis for several years, there is a definite risk of supervening carcinoma of the colon, a complication that may be difficult to recognize radiologically.

The etiology of ulcerative colitis is unknown. It is regarded as a systemic disease because of the frequently associated systemic manifestations, which include iritis, arthritis, erythema nodosum, and pyoderma gangrenosum.

The treatment depends upon the stage of the disease and the extent of involvement. Steroids, blood transfusions, and supportive measures are necessary in the acute fulminating phase of the disease. A low-residue diet, Azulfidine, steroids, and sometimes psychiatric care are useful during the chronic indolent phase of ulcerative colitis. Surgery is advised when the patient has perforation of the colon, is exsanguinating from colonic bleeding, has toxic megacolon, or is unresponsive to medical management. Many gastroenterologists and surgeons advise colectomy to eliminate the very substantial risk of carcinoma of the colon.

At this time *Clotilde* is being managed medically. She seems to be doing only fairly well. Her parents have been informed of the risk of carcinoma, and we suspect that they will agree to total colectomy in the near future.

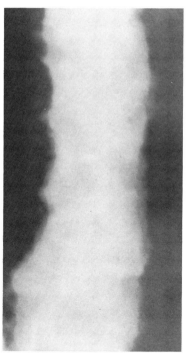

Figure 107. Clotilde, spot film

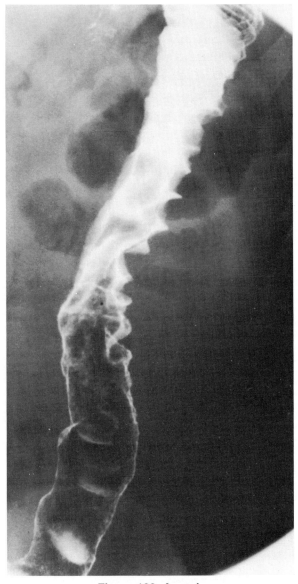

Figure 108. Anna L.

Anna Larson is a pale 5 year old girl with symptoms of coryza, diarrhea, and the recent onset of blood in her stools. Her pediatrician suspected inflammatory bowel disease and requested an air-contrast barium enema, one film of which is presented here. Given the further information that Anna's renal profile indicated deteriorating kidney function, can you propose a diagnosis?

ANSWER

The radiograph from the barium enema shows spasm and "thumb printing," or thick indentations of the colonic wall. In this case, the "thumb printing" is due to intramural hemorrhage that distorts the normal colonic contour. Now note the tiny ulcerations, which you can see as white dots projecting from colonic lumen. Colonic ulcerations and intramural hemorrhage in a child with a rising blood urea nitrogen (BUN) should lead you to consider the hemolytic-uremic syndrome. Children with this syndrome have a microangiopathic hemolytic anemia, acute renal insufficiency, and, about 20 per cent of the time, colitis with gastrointestinal bleeding. Many children also have other problems such as coma, confusion, or seizures. The diagnosis is based on the combination of microangiopathic hemolysis and renal impairment. Treatment includes dialysis and other supportive measures.

TWO NEWBORN BABIES WITH FEEDING DIFFICULTY

Baby Boy Neville St. Clair, 2 days
old, was the product of a normal full-
term pregnancy. Shortly after birth,
his abdomen became distended, and
mucous secretions accumulated
about his mouth. He regurgitated his
first and only feeding. The pediatric
intern was unable to pass a nasogastric tube into the stomach. He made
a presumptive diagnosis, and it was
confirmed by the radiographs of the
chest (Figs. 109 and 110), which
were obtained after 1 ml. of contrast
material (oily Dionosil) was injected
into the esophageal pouch through
the tube.

Review of these radiographs established the diagnosis and treatment was initiated.

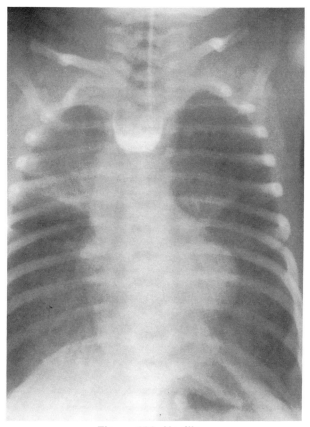

Figure 109. Neville

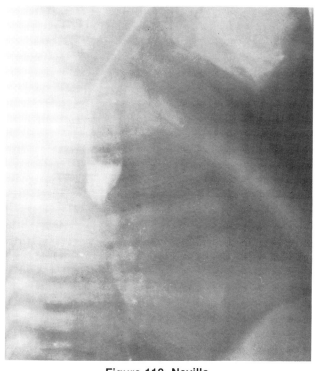

Figure 110. Neville

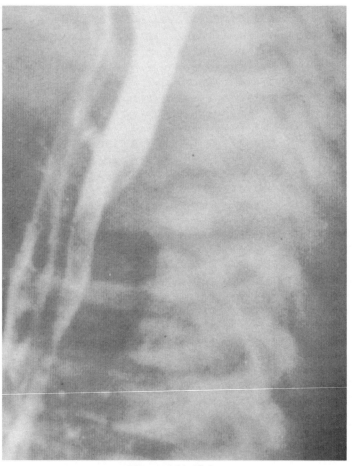

Figure 111. Kate

Baby Girl Kate Whitney was the product of a normal pregnancy and delivery. Her physical examination at birth was negative. However, feedings were initiated with great difficulty because each feeding caused coughing, choking, and cyanosis. A chest radiograph in the newborn nursery suggested pneumonia. The radiologist reviewed the history with the pediatricians and suggested an esophagogram (Fig. 111).

ANSWERS

Baby Boy Neville St. Clair's radiographs demonstrate that the esophagus is dilated and ends in a blind pouch. The air in the stomach (both views) indicates that there must be a connection between the outside atmosphere and the gastrointestinal tract. Since the proximal esophagus is atretic, there must be a distal tracheoesophageal fistula. This is the most common form of the esophageal atresia–tracheoesophageal fistula complex.

Notice that there are bilateral upper lobe infiltrates. *Neville* was unable to swallow his saliva or his first feeding, resulting in aspiration of both.

Neville was started on antibiotic therapy, and then surgery was performed. The distal tracheoesophageal fistula was ligated, and the two esophageal segments were anastomosed.

Had *Neville* been too ill to tolerate a primary anastomosis, a gastrostomy would have been performed for decompression of the gastrointestinal tract and for feeding. Then, when his condition was stable, the definitive surgery would have been performed.

As it was, *Neville* did well following surgery. When he was 10 months old, a barium swallow showed minimal narrowing at the level of the anastomosis of the two portions of the esophagus and abnormal peristalsis in the middle third of the esophagus.

When *Baby Girl Kate Whitney* was seen by her pediatrician, it was not clear whether she was aspirating her feedings because of incoordinated swallowing or had a tracheoesophageal fistula. (Esophageal atresia had been ruled out by passing a nasogastric tube into the stomach.) A contrast study (Fig. 111) demonstrated a fistulous communication low in the neck, between the trachea and esophagus. (Barium was not used because the radiologist was afraid that if it was aspirated or there was a "T-E" fistula, barium might enter the lungs. Oily Dionosil was used—the same agent used for bronchograms.)

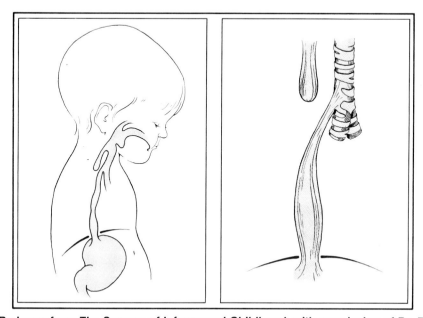

Figure 112. (Redrawn from *The Surgery of Infancy and Childhood,* with permission of Dr. Robert Gross)

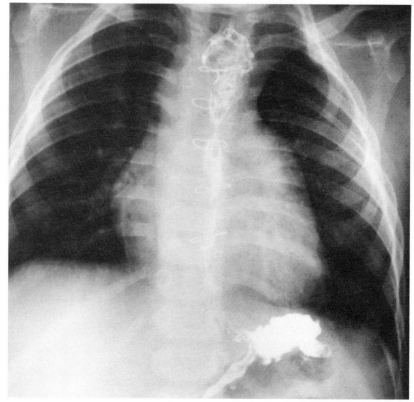

Figure 113.

Kate has an isolated tracheoesophageal fistula. The fistula was ligated and divided. Recovery was prompt, and the child had no further difficulties.

One of the more common delayed complications of the surgical repair of tracheoesophageal fistula is the development of a narrowed segment at the site of the anastomosis of the proximal esophagus to the distal esophagus. In the case illustrated in Figure 113, an apricot is lodged in the dilated esophagus just above the anastomotic site. This was removed at endoscopy, and the narrowed area was dilated.

Max Wilms, age 6 years, complained of progressive difficulty swallowing all foods, but especially solids.

This single spot radiograph obtained during fluoroscopy for *Max Wilms'* barium esophagogram shows a localized constriction in the upper esophagus. This narrowing was a consistent finding throughout the study. Do you have a diagnosis?

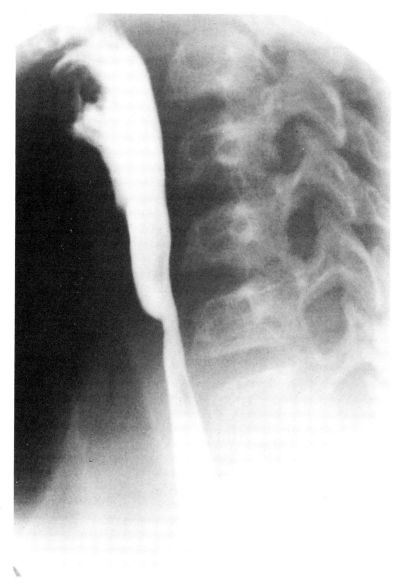

Figure 114. Max Wilms

ANSWER

Max Wilms has an iris-type diaphragm, or web, of the esophagus. These webs, which are quite uncommon, are frequently difficult to visualize on an esophagogram, and the diagnosis may be delayed for years. In this case, endoscopy proved the roentgenographic diagnosis, and dilation was effective in treating *Max's* swallowing disorder.

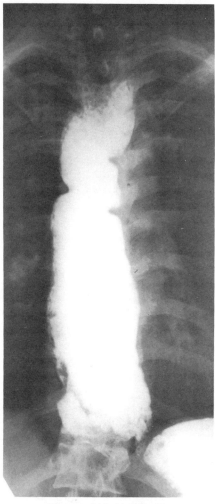

Figure 115. V. Mikulicz

Von Mikulicz is an adolescent boy who has a great deal of difficulty swallowing. What are the radiographic findings on his esophagogram, which is illustrated here?

ANSWER

Notice on this radiograph, which was obtained while the child was standing upright, that almost the entire esophagus is filled, that the esophagus is dilated, and that there is a very smooth tapering of the esophagus at the gastroesophageal junction. Fluoroscopy was performed while our patient swallowed his barium meal, and markedly reduced peristalsis was observed.

The condition with which this boy is afflicted is called achalasia. The term itself means "absence of relaxation," and refers to the physiologic abnormality of the esophagus at the gastroesophageal junction. The esophagus of patients with achalasia can become so dilated that aspiration with pneumonia, malnutrition, vomiting, and fetor oris (bad breath) may develop.

Treatment programs for this disease have included balloon dilation of the esophagogastric junction as well as the Heller (no relation to the Heller who is co-author of this book!) procedure, a myotomy of the esophageal muscle down to the submucosa at the level of the narrowing.

AN INFANT WITH CONTINUOUS PURULENT DISCHARGE FROM THE LEFT NOSTRIL

John Openshaw is an infant who had a chronic purulent discharge from the left nostril, which seemed to be plugged. The pediatrician suspected that the child had unilateral choanal atresia because he was unable to pass a catheter through the left nostril down to the level of the oropharynx. *John* was referred to the Radiology Department for a "choanogram."

For this procedure, the patient was placed in the supine position and immobilized by a sheet that was elaborately wrapped around him (mummification); this is really quite comfortable. The radiologist then passed a radiopaque catheter into the right nostril and docu-

mented its patency with a lateral radiograph of the nasopharynx and oropharynx (Fig. 116).

A catheter was then introduced into the left nostril, where it met total obstruction. The secretions that had accumulated in the nostril were removed and the radiologist tried again, with no success. He then injected 3 ml. of oily Dionosil through the catheter, and the technologist obtained three views of the area: the lateral view (Fig. 117), the AP view (Fig. 118), and the base view (Fig. 119). X-ray computed tomography (not illustrated) was also performed.

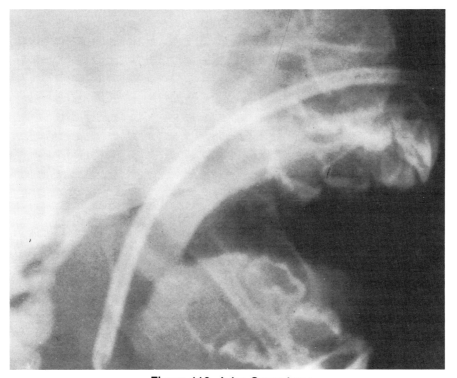

Figure 116. John Openshaw

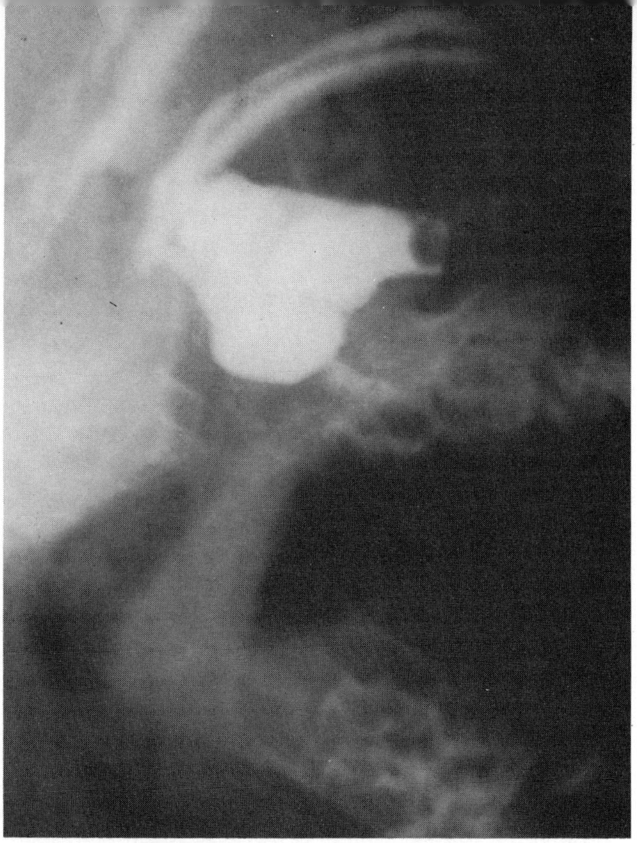

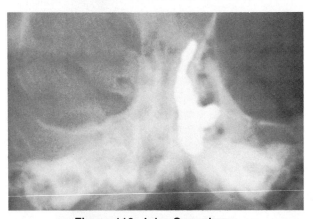

Figure 117. John Openshaw

ANSWER

John Openshaw's radiographs demonstrated that there is a total obstruction of the left choana (posterior naris). The obstruction is caused by a membranous or bony partition that closes the nasal airway above the posterior end of the hard palate. This condition may be unilateral or bilateral and is known as choanal atresia.

Bilateral choanal atresia is especially serious in the newborn because it may take days for the baby to learn mouth-breathing. Because of the dependency on nasal breathing, the newborn may die of asphyxia if choanal atresia is not recognized. Some babies with bilateral choanal atresia will quickly learn to breathe through the mouth, but upon feeding, they will become cyanotic and dyspneic. Unilateral choanal atresia is not as serious a condition in the newborn period. It usually is not recognized until the child is evaluated for unilateral nasal obstruction or abnormal quality of the voice.

Treatment of bilateral choanal atresia is initiated by maintenance of an oral airway. The child may be fed with a stomach tube or medicine dropper until he learns to suck and breathe alternately. If the obstruction is caused by a membrane, it may be resected, utilizing an anterior nasal approach. A bony partition causing obstruction requires a transpalatal approach and removal of the obstruction. The main postoperative problem is restenosis of the posterior choanae.

No definitive surgery is planned at the present time for *John*. The plan is to encourage the mother to keep the nose clean of accumulated secretions, and if the child's voice does not have an abnormal quality, surgery will be delayed until the baby is older, or it may be omitted altogether.

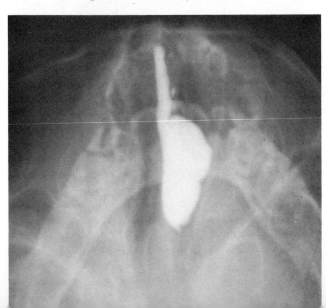

Figure 118. John Openshaw

Figure 119. John Openshaw

TWO NEWBORN BABIES WITH INCREASING ABDOMINAL DISTENTION AND NO STOOLS

Baby Girl Mary Sutherland was less than 12 hours old when her abdomen began to appear distended. At 20 hours she began to vomit greenish material. At the end of her first day no meconium had yet been passed.

The initial physical examination at the time of delivery showed nothing abnormal. The baby was re-examined at 12 hours because the nurses in the newborn nursery were concerned about the abdominal distention. (A smart house officer can learn a lot of pediatrics from the nursing staff. If communication lines are in good working order, the nurses will inform him of small problems before they become big problems and of big problems before they become disasters.) The house officer found *Baby Girl Sutherland* unchanged since his initial physical examination, except that her abdomen was protuberant and her flanks bulged. He could feel no abdominal masses.

The baby was re-examined at 24 hours because of vomiting, lack of stools, and persistent abdominal distention. Included in the workup was a supine view of the chest and abdomen (Fig. 120).

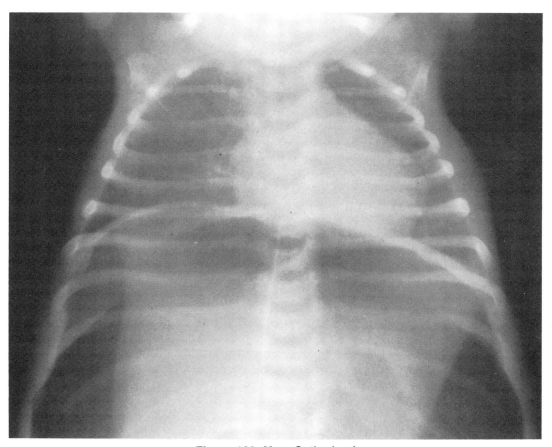

Figure 120. Mary Sutherland

Baby Boy Hosmer Angel appeared to be normal at birth. Like *Baby Girl Mary Sutherland*, he developed abdominal distention and passed no meconium during the first day of life. The baby began to appear ill, with pallor and increased respiratory rate. A "sepsis workup" (culture of the blood, urine, cerebrospinal fluid, and tracheal aspirate, with Gram stain to help identify any bacteria) was done. An AP view of the abdomen (Fig. 121) was obtained.

The radiologists interpreted this view of the abdomen as showing distended loops of bowel with an especially distended portion of the gut in the right lower quadrant in the region where the cecum would be expected to be. (In babies, it is very hard to differentiate small bowel from colon by a plain radiograph. The only way to be certain is to perform a contrast enema.) The radiologists were concerned about a collection of gas bubbles in the right lower quadrant and speculated that this was an abscess. It was suggested that the other areas of bowel were distended on the basis of ileus secondary to obstruction by the abscess. The differential diagnosis included a cecal perforation and appendicitis with periappendiceal abscess, which is rare in newborn full-term infants.

Baby Boy Hosmer was operated upon, and at surgery the cecum was found to be grossly distended. There were two pinpoint perforations from which bowel contents had contaminated the peritoneal cavity near the cecum. A cecostomy was done to decompress the cecum, and the baby was treated with antibiotics.

It is very rare for a newborn baby to "blow out" the cecum, but when it occurs a second associated diagnosis should come to mind. Which further measures should be taken?

Figure 121. Hosmer Angel

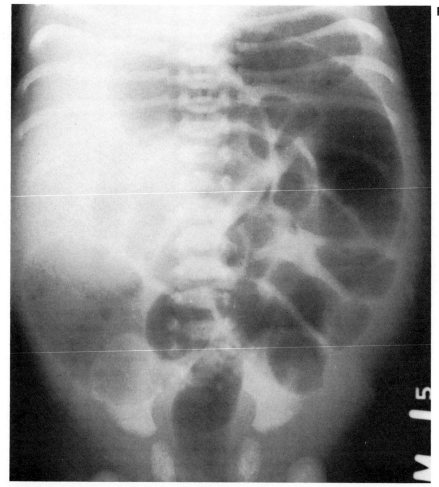

ANSWERS

The pediatric house officer caring for *Baby Girl Sutherland* did not believe the report of free air in the peritoneal cavity that was called to him in the newborn nursery from the Radiology Department. So, he descended to the subterranean depths of the hospital to the Pediatric Radiology Department and reviewed the radiographs with the pediatric radiologists. It was pointed out that the linear shadow projected over the right side of the lower thoracic vertebral bodies was the falciform ligament. This extends from the diaphragm and anterior abdominal wall to the caudal edge of the liver and, being water-dense, can't be seen unless outlined by air. Furthermore, the large mass of air in the peritoneal cavity forms an oval shape on the supine radiograph as it outlines the edge of the peritoneal cavity (Fig. 120).

To expedite the surgery and to convince the skeptical, an abdominal radiograph in the upright position was taken, which also showed the falciform ligament (Fig. 122, arrow). In addition, the spleen and liver have fallen away from the diaphragm, and the superior portion of the peritoneal cavity is filled with air.

At surgery, an ileal stenosis with perforation was found; this was resected, and an end-to-end anastomosis was performed. The etiology of the stenosis was not determined, but the possibility of an intrauterine bowel infarction possibly caused by a local volvulus was raised. *Baby Girl Sutherland* recovered promptly from her surgery and has subsequently gone home. She seems well on return visits to the Outpatient Department.

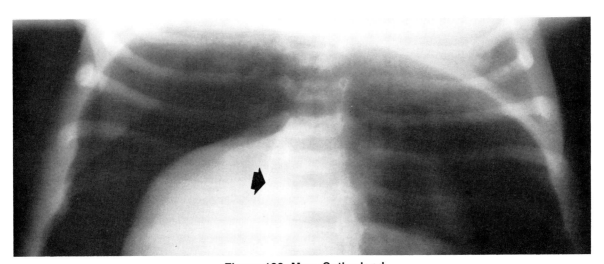

Figure 122. Mary Sutherland

Baby Boy Hosmer Angel soon regained his birth weight. His cecostomy functioned well, and he seemed to thrive in the nursery.

It is well known that in adults an obstruction in the colon, either inflammatory or neoplastic, may present clinically as cecal perforation. Diverticulitis and carcinoma of the colon don't occur in the newborn, but another condition does, and the workup for this includes a barium enema (Figs. 123 and 124).

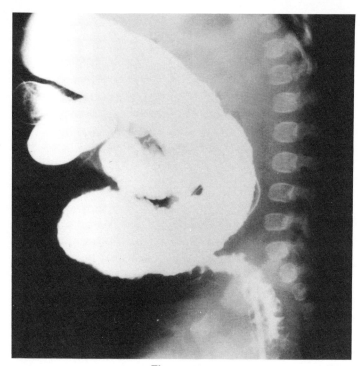

Figure 123.

The lateral (Fig. 123) and AP (Fig. 124) projections demonstrate a contracted segment of lower sigmoid colon (arrow). Above the site of the narrowing, the colon displays bizarre irregular contractions with a saw-toothed appearance. These are the radiologic findings of Hirschsprung's disease.

In this condition, the parasympathetic innervation of the affected portion of the colon including the ganglion cells is absent. The parasympathetic system is responsible for the propulsive contractility of the colon. When the ganglion cells of the myenteric plexus are absent, a physiologic obstruction occurs, with dilation of the bowel proximal to the area of absent ganglion cells. The barium enema shows a contracted distal segment, the aganglionic bowel, and a "transition zone" above which the normal but obstructed colon is dilated. The diagnosis is proved by rectal biopsy, which shows absence of the ganglion cells.

The initial treatment for this condition is decompressive colostomy or cecostomy proximal to the aganglionic segment. This diverts the fecal stream and prevents the complication of enterocolitis. The aim of surgery is to reconstitute normal function of the colon. This is performed by removing the functionally obstructing segment of the colon or rerouting the fecal stream so as to anastomose normal colon to the anus.

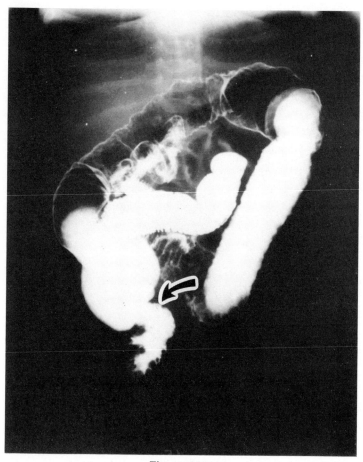

Figure 124.

THE CASE OF THE MISSING ANUS

Baby Boy Jabez Wilson was discovered to have entered this world incompletely equipped. In place of an anus he had a small dimple that didn't communicate with the large bowel within—in other words, an imperforate anus. The workup for this included a supine radiograph of the abdomen and chest (Fig. 125). The metallic density is an umbilical cord clamp. The study shows absence of gas in the rectum and a normal lumbar spine and sacrum.

The latter finding may help to distinguish the two principal types of imperforate anus: high and low. Spine abnormalities are common with the high anomaly but are infrequent with the low.

In the high anomaly, the rectal pouch ends above the pelvic floor (actually the levator ani muscles). A fistula usually is present, extending from the rectum to the posterior urethra or bladder in boys and to the vagina in girls. This high anomaly is treated initially by a colostomy, followed one to two years later by an exacting abdominoperineal operation. The fistula is divided and the distal colon is pulled through the pelvic

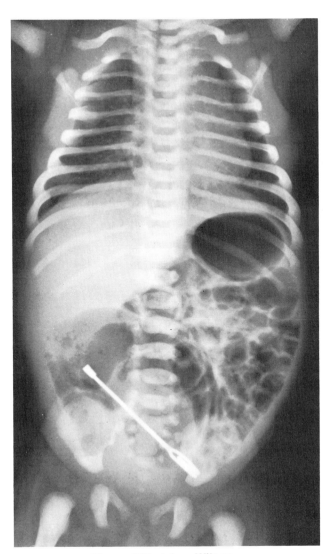

Figure 125. Jabez Wilson

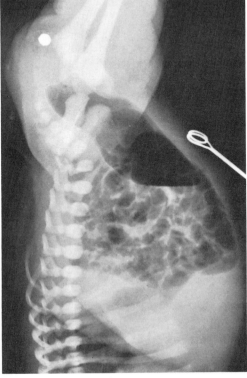

Figure 126. Jabez Wilson

floor in an attempt to establish as normal a relationship as possible of the terminal colon to the levator ani sling. Finally the pouch is attached at the anal dimple, and an opening is made.

In the low anomaly the rectum passes normally through the levator ani sling. Repair is simpler and is usually done shortly after birth, using only a perineal approach. When fistulas occur they are to the perineum, the base of the scrotum, or the vestibule.

For practical purposes, the clinical differentiation of high and low anomalies may be made by determining the site of the fistula, if present. Of course, a major concern is the distance between the blind rectal pouch and the anal dimple. The classic way to show this has been an "upside-down view" (Figs. 126 and 127).

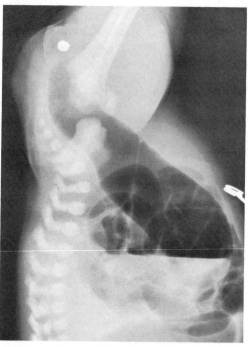

Figure 127. Jabez Wilson

The theory is that the gas in the colon will seek the highest level. If a marker is placed on the anal dimple and a true lateral view of the pelvis is obtained with the baby held upside down, a close approximation of the distance between the blind rectal pouch and the anal dimple may be possible. This was done with *Baby Boy Jabez Wilson* (Fig. 126). At 14 hours after birth there was a 2 cm. separation between the distal bowel gas and anal dimple. Fortunately, another radiograph (Fig. 127) taken 22 hours after birth shows the separation to be less than 1 cm. The implication from this second film is that this is a low anomaly and repair *can* be performed using the much simpler perineal approach. Why was the distance greater 14 hours after birth? Presumably the swallowed air had not yet reached the rectum or had not displaced the meconium already there.

Most pediatric radiologists have learned to interpret the upside-down view with caution or to recommend that it not be obtained at all, since at times it may not accurately reflect the anatomy. A low anomaly may appear to be high, as it did on the 14 hour film of *Baby Boy Wilson*, or a high anomaly may appear to be low if the film is made as the infant strains vigorously. Clinical and radiographic assessment of the site of the fistula more reliably differentiates high and low anomalies.

Jabez Wilson's surgery was successful, and he has had an uneventful childhood.

Any idea of the derivation of the patients' names?

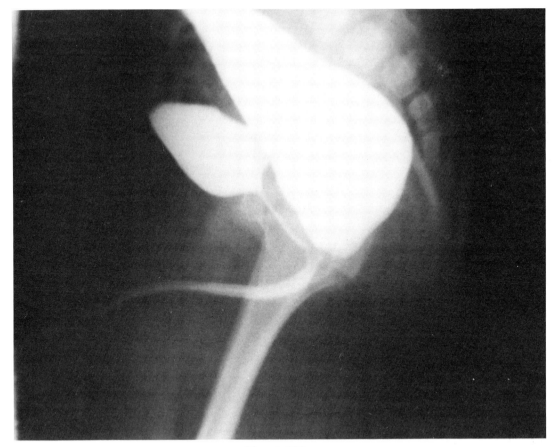

Figure 128.

By the way, Thomas Hodgkin died in Jaffa, Israel, in 1866 of dysentery while on a trip with Sir Moses Montefiore.

This male baby with imperforate anus (Fig. 128) has a fistula between the rectum and the prostatic urethra. The bladder was catheterized and filled with diluted water-soluble contrast material. When the baby urinated, contrast passed through the fistula and opacified the colon.

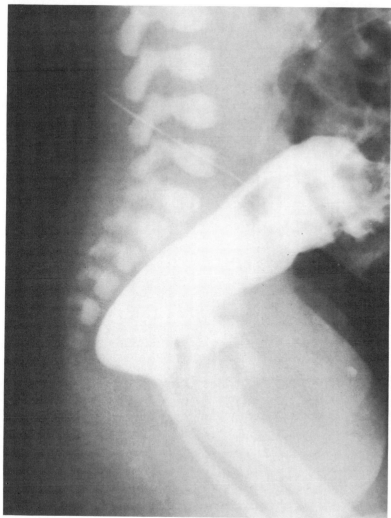

Figure 129.

The radiograph illustrated in Figure 129 was obtained in a newborn baby with a single opening on the perineum. In this study, contrast was injected into this orifice. Now for the questions! Which organs are opacified? What is the name of this anomaly? In what group of animals is this the normal state of affairs?

ANSWER

Our radiograph shows opacification of the rectum and sigmoid colon. In addition, contrast is seen anterior to the rectum and colon in the bladder and vagina. This is the typical appearance of one type of cloacal anomaly, which is caused by failure of the cloaca to be divided by the urorectal septum. Complex anomalies of the genitourinary tract are associated with this lesion in humans; however, this is the normal state in birds!

Urgent surgical correction is necessary.

THE CASE OF THE DOUBLE BUBBLE

Baby Girl Culverton Smith, 4 days old, had had bilious vomiting since birth and was quite dehydrated.

The physical examination did not reveal the cause of the vomiting. A supine AP radiograph of the abdomen (Fig. 130) demonstrated only a small amount of air in the stomach. A nasogastric tube was placed in the stomach, and gastric contents were aspirated. Then air was injected into the stomach and supine and upright views were obtained (Fig. 131 and 132).

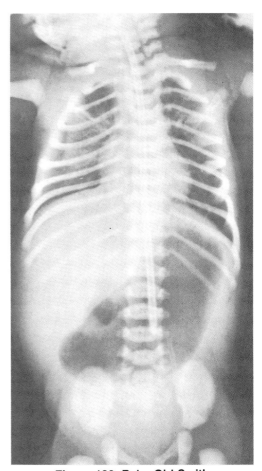

Figure 130. Baby Girl Smith

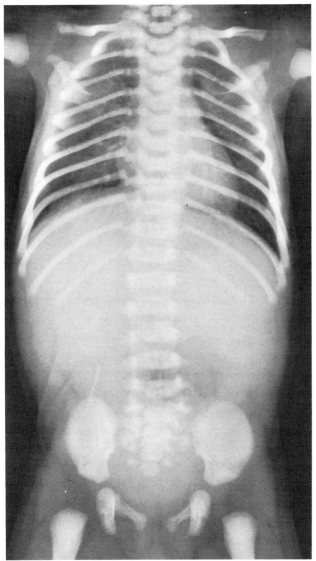

Figure 131. Baby Girl Smith

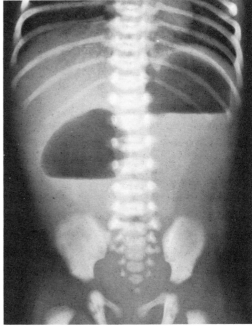

Figure 132. Baby Girl Smith

ANSWER

Air as contrast material is not emphasized as much as the more expensive water-soluble contrast agents (Gastrografin, Renografin) or old reliable barium. Actually, the upright view of the abdomen with air injected into the stomach yields all the information necessary without the risk of the other materials. (The water-soluble contrast materials should almost never be given by mouth to babies. Because of their hyperosmolarity, water is drawn into the small bowel and the baby becomes profoundly dehydrated.) Barium may be used, but if the baby vomits, he may have trouble clearing the vomitus from the facial area and may aspirate barium into the lungs. Air in moderate amounts is diagnostic; it is also safe, readily available, and inexpensive.

The analysis of the upright radiograph shows two air-fluid interfaces. The one to the left of the spine is in the stomach. Review of the supine abdominal view shows air in the stomach and duodenum but not further along in the small bowel. The air-fluid interface to the right of the spine ought to be in the duodenum, and there should be an obstruction *distal* to the ampulla of Vater because of the bilious character of the vomitus.

This radiologic pattern is called the "double bubble sign," and it is seen in only a few conditions. At surgery *Culverton Smith* had duodenal atresia, but the "double bubble sign" is also seen in annular pancreas, in which the duodenal obstruction is caused by extrinsic compression. Much more commonly the sign is seen with midgut volvulus. Intrinsic obstruction of the duodenum may also occur if there is severe duodenal stenosis.

The differentiation of the several possibilities mentioned above can be aided by looking at the corners of the radiograph. For example, it is known that duodenal atresia is associated with Down's syndrome. If the pelvis shows flared iliac wings and flattened acetabular roofs, duodenal atresia should be at the top of the diagnostic list because the patient is likely to have Down's syndrome (this pelvis is normal). Likewise, if a barium enema shows a malposition of the cecum, malrotation with midgut volvulus should be diagnosis *numero uno.*

The problem, in fact, is a surgical one, but the aim of the radiologist is to narrow the possible causes so that the surgeon will have some idea of what to expect and will be able to plan accordingly. This child was successfully operated upon for duodenal atresia.

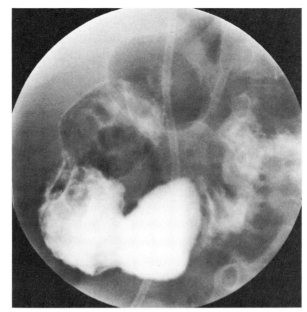

Enoch Drebber is a newborn with bilious vomiting.

Figure 133. Enoch Drebber

ANSWER

The radiograph presented here is one of several obtained during an upper gastrointestinal examination. Note the almost complete obstruction at the junction of the second and third portions of the duodenum. This obstruction is caused by a transverse diaphragm (arrow) with only a few fenestrations that permit some forward progress of the barium. The diaphragm is pushed forward by gastric and duodenal secretions and eventually assumes the configuration termed "wind sock" diaphragm. The treatment of a duodenal web is surgical excision to relieve the obstruction.

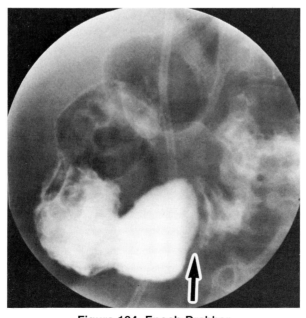

Figure 134. Enoch Drebber

THREE TEENAGERS: ONE WITH VOMITING, ONE WITH RIGHT LOWER QUADRANT ABDOMINAL PAIN, AND ONE WITH BRIGHT RED RECTAL BLEEDING

Honoria Westphail is a 13 year old girl who was admitted to the hospital because of vomiting, weight loss, and gradually shortening hair braids. The physical examination revealed a slender girl with a somewhat malnourished appearance. There was a mass in the left upper quadrant of the abdomen. A "scout" radiograph of the abdomen (Fig. 135) and an upper gastrointestinal series were performed.

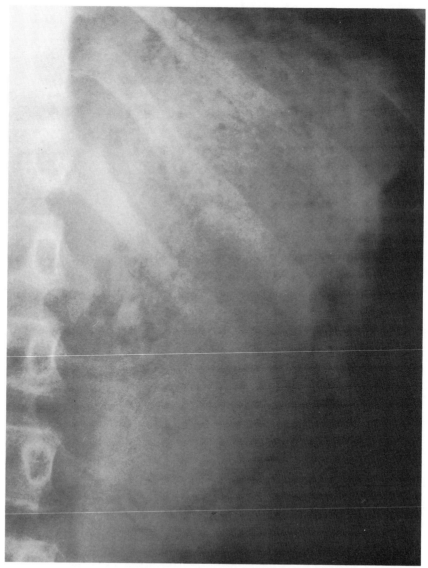

Figure 135. Honoria Westphail

Figure 136. Grimesby Roylott

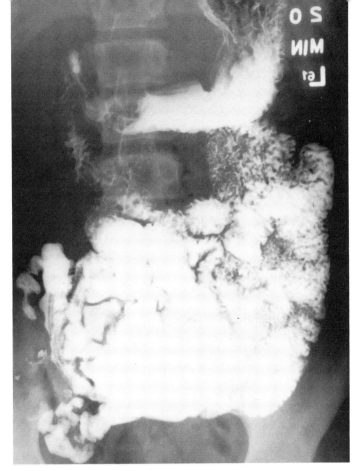

Grimesby Roylott, a 15 year old boy from a rural Appalachian area, was referred to the Radiology Department for an upper gastrointestinal series and small bowel follow-through (Fig. 136) because of cramping, intermittent right lower quadrant abdominal pain. He denied all other symptoms and did not appear ill. The physical examination was normal.

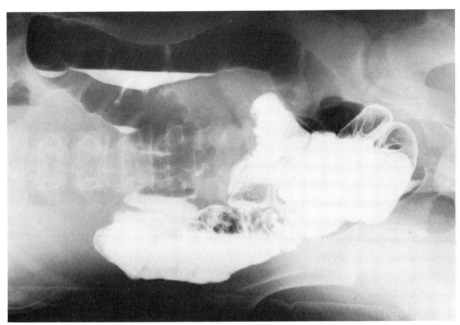

Figure 137. Percy Armitage

Percy Armitage is a 13 year old schoolboy from the Eastern Shore of Maryland. He was completely well except that one day he noticed bright red blood in the toilet after a bowel movement. His pediatrician could find no cause for the bleeding and referred the child to a radiologist for an air contrast barium enema. (Figure 137 is a right lateral decubitus radiograph.)

ANSWERS

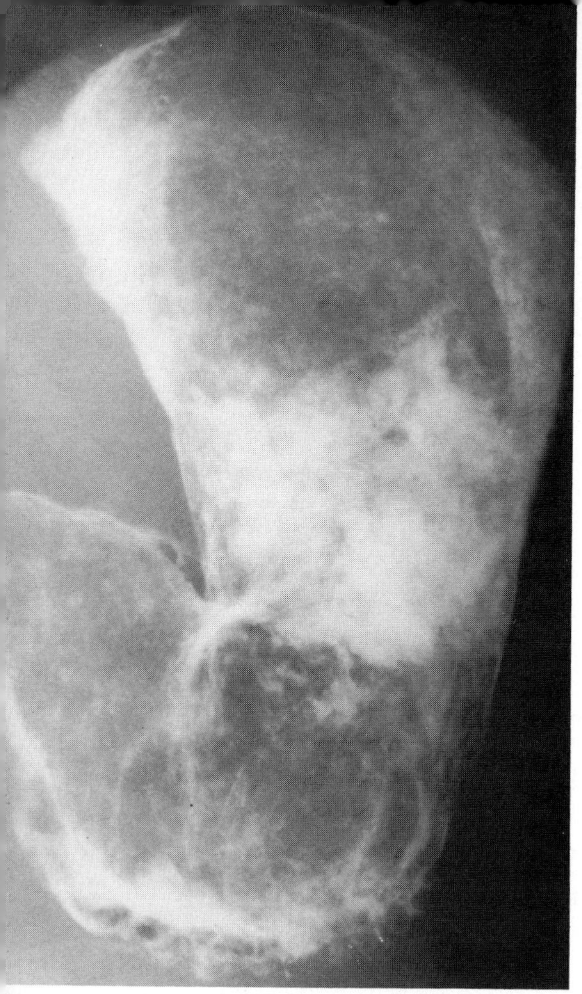

Figure 138. Honoria Westphail

Honoria Westphail was a somewhat anxious girl with the strange habit of eating her own hair—trichophagia. Figure 135 shows the stomach filled with radiolucent material. After several mouthfuls of barium were swallowed, a trichobezoar was outlined by the barium that flowed around it (Fig. 138).

The treatment for a trichobezoar is gastrotomy and removal of the mass. If the trichobezoar extends into the small bowel, it must also be removed from that area to prevent obstruction.

This condition usually occurs in teenage girls who are emotionally disturbed. *Honoria* has been undergoing psychotherapy while recovering from her surgery. It is expected that this therapy will be continued on an outpatient basis after her discharge from the hospital.

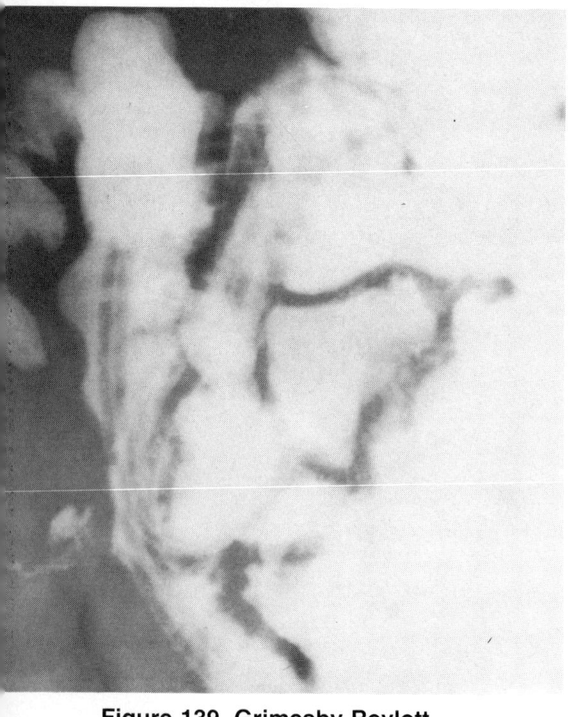

Figure 139. Grimesby Roylott

Grimesby Roylott unknowingly brought a few of his friends with him for a free upper gastrointestinal series. Look closely at the right lower quadrant region and you will see several long cylindrical objects with white streaks running down their middles. These roundworms, *Ascaris lumbricoides,* are making their home in *Grimesby's* small bowel and are ingesting the barium their host has provided. The white streak outlines the gastrointestinal tract of the worm (normal so far as we can tell).

Grimesby was treated with piperazine, the drug of choice for ascariasis. We are not certain that his symptoms were related to the worms, because frequently ascariasis is asymptomatic. At any rate, since treatment *Grimesby* says he feels better.

Percy did not like his preparation for the air contrast barium enema, which consisted of several days of a clear liquid diet, a cathartic, and an enema, but the result was a moderately clean colon in which the polyp and its stalk in the descending colon were clearly identified, free of obscuring feces. Several other shadows were thought to be feces rather than polyps, a distinction difficult to make if the colon is not well prepared.

The radiologist thought that the lesion identified was a juvenile polyp (Fig. 140), although usually such polyps are seen in younger children around the age of 5. Juvenile polyps are not true polyps but are composed largely of fibrous tissue with little overlying epithelium. They are thought to arise from chronic inflammation, perhaps with obstruction of the mucous glands. The juvenile polyps may have a long stalk or a sessile, mushroom-like appearance with a broad base attached to the colonic wall. The force of peristalsis may cause a juvenile polyp to be the lead point of an intussusception. Alternatively, the fecal stream may erode the polyp and cause rectal bleeding.

Juvenile polyps do not resemble the adenomatous polyps of adulthood. They do not become malignant. If left alone, they will slough spontaneously. Surgery is indicated, however, if a juvenile polyp causes excessive bleeding, if it prolapses through the anus, or if it can be shown that the polyp is the lead point of an intussusception.

The most important lesion to exclude in the differential diagnosis of polypoid lesions in children is the adenomatous polyp of familial polyposis. Since one or more of these very numerous polyps will ultimately become malignant, colectomy must be considered. The radiologist and the pediatrician questioned *Percy's* mother about her health and that of her husband, looking for any evidence of a history of familial polyposis or carcinoma of the colon. Because familial polyposis is inherited as a mendelian dominant trait, and because his parents are normal, it would be relatively unlikely that *Percy* has familial polyposis (see Fig. 141).

Other conditions that were considered are the Peutz-Jeghers form of intestinal polyposis. This condition is accompanied by melanin spots around the mouth and on the buccal mucosa (see Fig. 142). These lesions were not found on *Percy*. Gardner's syndrome (multiple polyposis with sebaceous cysts and bone tumors) was dismissed because the last two findings weren't present.

The child was periodically checked to be certain that he did not become anemic owing to excessive bleeding. He has had no further bleeding, so the polyp has probably spontaneously sloughed.

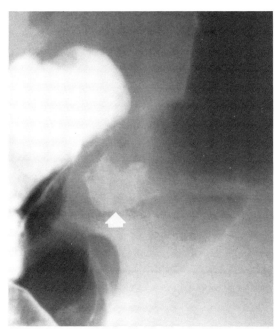

Figure 140. Percy Armitage

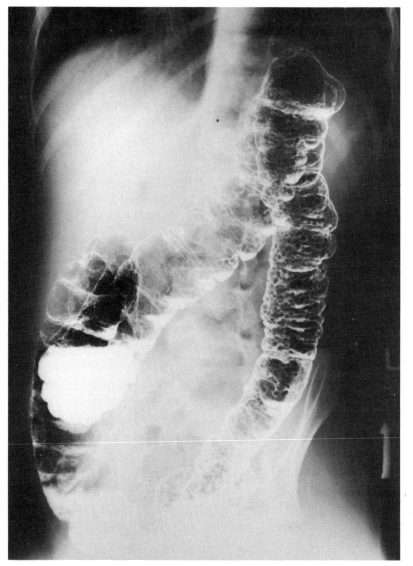

Figure 141.

Patients with familial polyposis are detected because of anemia, rectal bleeding, or a family history of the disease, which is inherited as an autosomal dominant trait. These patients should have a prophylactic colectomy, because cancer of the colon invariably develops unless surgery is performed. This radiograph (Fig. 141) from the barium enema performed in a child with familial polyposis shows tiny polyps that stud the mucosa.

Patients with Peutz-Jeghers syndrome, also inherited as an autosomal dominant trait, have hamartomatous polyps of the small bowel (and occasionally the stomach and colon) and the previously mentioned melanin pigment spots about the mouth, the buccal mucosa, and the anus. It is important to recall that there is an increased incidence of carcinoma of the stomach, duodenum, and ileum in patients with the Peutz-Jeghers syndrome, as well as an increased incidence of bowel obstruction. This radiograph from an upper gastrointestinal series (Fig. 142) shows irregular filling defects, which represent a polypoid mass in the duodenum of a child with Peutz-Jeghers syndrome.

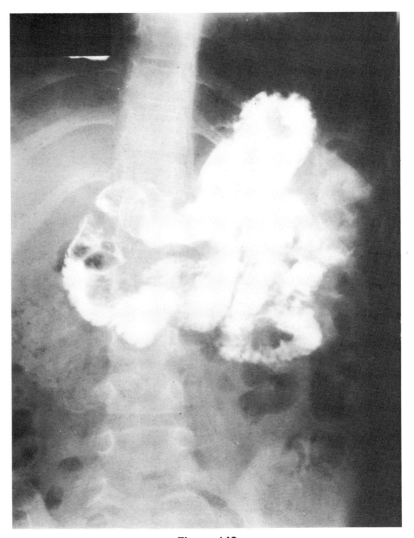

Figure 142.

A NEWBORN WITH BOWEL OBSTRUCTION

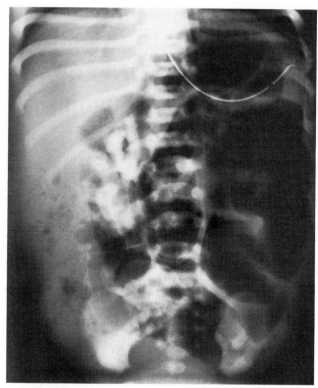

Figure 143. Watson

The radiograph in Figure 143 was obtained because of bilious vomiting and abdominal distention in a 24 hour old baby boy named **Watson**. During this time, the baby had not passed any meconium, and it was thought that he had an intestinal obstruction at an unknown site. The possibilities included ileal or jejunal atresia, malrotation with volvulus or obstructing bands, Hirschsprung's disease, and meconium ileus.

The supine abdominal radiograph (Fig. 143) shows clearly distended loops of bowel in the left side of the abdomen. In the right lower quadrant of the abdomen, collections of gas are seen interspersed with soft tissue density material, in this case probably meconium (although gas in an abscess might have this appearance). Although this is not a finding that is absolutely specific, it is

seen when gas in the ileum is forced by peristaltic waves into meconium that is more viscid than normal. The thick, sticky meconium obstructs the ileum and is responsible for the bilious vomiting, abdominal distention, and failure to pass stools.

This condition is known as meconium ileus, and it is only one of the manifestations of cystic fibrosis (also known as mucoviscidosis). This disease is inherited as an autosomal recessive condition that affects the exocrine glands in varying degrees. The mucous secretions are excessively viscid. In the intestines, this causes the meconium to become tenacious and leads to a bowel obstruction. In the lungs, the bronchi become obstructed by the thick mucus, and atelectasis and infections occur. In the sinuses, obstructed mucous glands and polyps are found. Obstruction of the bile ducts causes biliary cirrhosis, while the pancreatic ducts are frequently obstructed and the exocrine pancreatic glands gradually degenerate and are replaced by connective tissue.

If the baby has meconium ileus, we can expect the colon to be unused and empty, that is, to have a microcolon appearance.

It has been shown that if water soluble contrast materials such as Gastrografin or Renografin are used in an enema, the hyperosmolarity of these agents will "pull" water into the gut and may cause the meconium to become more dispersed in the contrast agent mixture, causing relief of the obstruction.

This diagnostic and therapeutic treatment plan is not used if there are clinical signs of peritonitis, sepsis, or perforation of the intestine or if free air is seen on the preliminary views of the abdomen. It requires recognition that dehydration will occur and that careful control of intravenous fluids is necessary.

ANSWER

When it became clear that *Baby Boy Watson's* condition was stable and when additional films made it clear that he had none of the contraindications to contrast study, a Gastrografin enema was given. This showed the small diameter of the bowel characteristic of microcolon (Fig. 144). There was reflux into the terminal ileum, which also had a small caliber and an unused appearance. The more proximal gas-filled bowel was dilated, indicating that the bowel obstruction had not been relieved and was in either the jejunum or more proximal ileum. At this point, the baby expelled the Gastrografin, and it can be seen outlining his buttocks and back. The child was washed and put in a dry blanket so that he would not get cold, and the study was repeated several hours later (Fig. 145). At this point, pellets of meconium can be seen in the descending colon. The Gastrografin was refluxed into the ileum and, with continued reflux, finally reached the dilated small bowel, which is seen in the right lower quadrant of the abdomen. Soon afterward, *Baby Boy Watson* started to pass meconium. (The baby did not become dehydrated even with the extensive reflux because of the intravenous fluid therapy.)

Had the water-soluble enema not worked, surgery for removal of the meconium would have been necessary. Such surgery has considerable risk and only moderate success. If the bowel is not viable, the necrotic segments are resected.

This form of neonatal bowel obstruction does not have a good prognosis, but as of now *Baby Boy Watson* has been discharged from the hospital in satisfactory condition. The pulmonary complications of cystic fibrosis presumably will develop later in childhood.

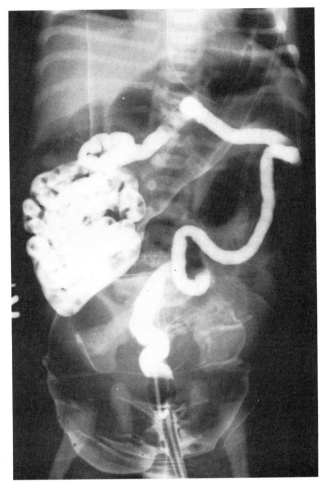

Figure 144. Watson

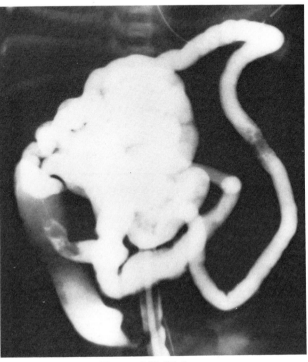

Figure 145. Watson

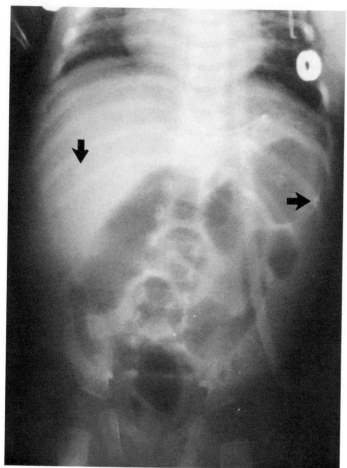

Figure 146.

If an intrauterine perforation of the intestines occurs with meconium spillage into the peritoneal cavity, punctate and plaque-like calcifications develop (Figs. 146 and 147, arrows). Two common causes of meconium peritonitis are an intrauterine vascular accident and meconium ileus. Although immediate surgical therapy may be required, in only a third of the cases is a site or cause of perforation ever found.

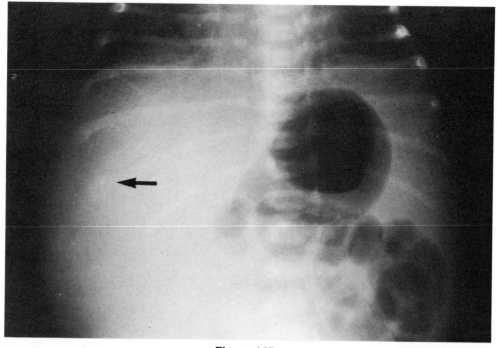

Figure 147.

Tobias Gregson, who was brought to the Emergency Room with vomiting and abdominal distention, had scrotal swelling on physical examination. His mother commented that this swelling had been present before and that it appeared and disappeared spontaneously.

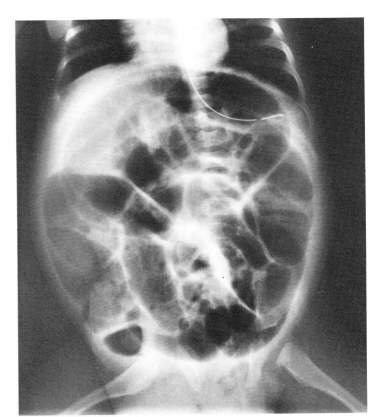

Figure 148. Tobias

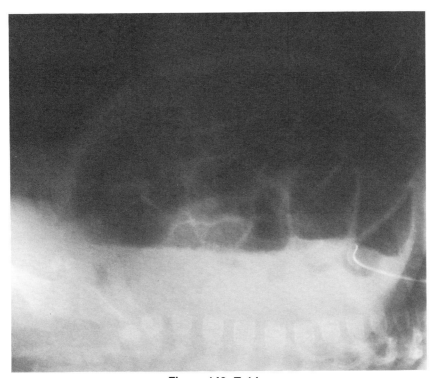

Figure 149. Tobias

ANSWER

As you examine *Tobias'* abdominal radiographs, don't forget to look carefully at the cross table lateral abdominal film. Of course you noticed the air-fluid levels, the extremely dilated small bowel, the absence of gas in the colon . . . and gas in the scrotum (arrow); well, that gas shouldn't be there! In fact, *Tobias Greg-son* has a small bowel obstruction, and it is caused by incarceration of a loop of small bowel in an inguinal hernia. By reading these radiographs correctly, you have detected an operative emergency, and prompt surgery will prevent ischemic necrosis of the incarcerated intestine.

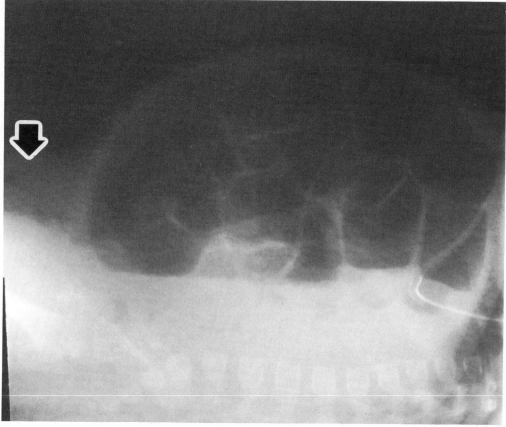

Figure 150. Tobias

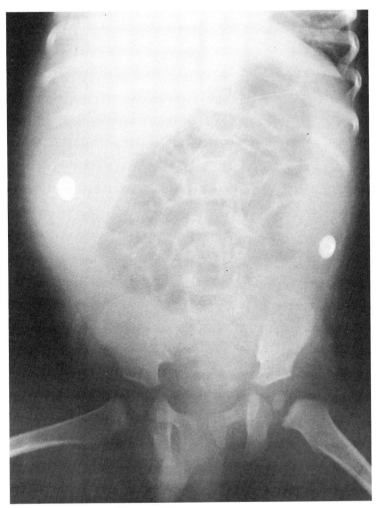

Vaughn Smith has *increasing* abdominal distention. What are the pertinent radiographic observations, and what is your conclusion?

Figure 151. Vaughn Smith

ANSWER

This is a supine, anteroposterior radiograph of *Vaughn Smith's* abdomen. First note the overall increased radiopacity present on this film. Do you also see that all the gas-filled bowel loops are, in fact, clustered in the center of the abdomen? Even the ascending colon is in more of a medial position than normal. The importance of the above observations is that they permit the recognition of free fluid in the peritoneal cavity. Un-

fortunately, the radiograph won't distinguish the causes, such as pus, urine, or even peritoneal dialysate. Although the findings on this particular film shout out to you that some sort of fluid is present, in many instances that is not the case. What is the best imaging modality available to detect small amounts of peritoneal fluid? If you said ultrasound, you're absolutely correct!

THE ADVENTURE OF THE DIRTY STOVE

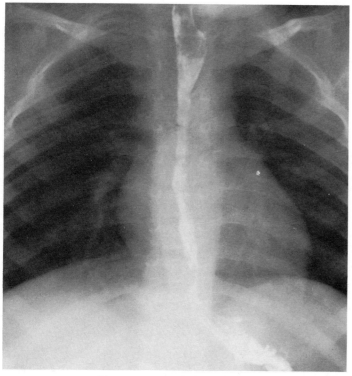

Figure 152. James Moriarty

James Moriarty, a 2 year old boy, was seen three weeks ago by his doctor because of coughing, vomiting, and inability to handle oral secretions for one day.

The doctor examined the boy at that time and diagnosed aphthous stomatitis, or canker sores. He prescribed aspirin and a mouthwash for relief of symptoms.

The day before these radiographs (Figs. 152 and 153) were obtained, *James* refused to swallow anything, including his saliva. The child was admitted to the hospital, and this barium swallow was performed. It was difficult for the boy to swallow because of pain. The radiologist, one S. Holmes, suggested that Mrs. Moriarty had recently been cleaning her stove, or possibly her sink, toilet, or bathtub. Why would Dr. Holmes make that suggestion?

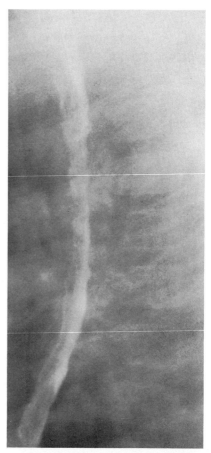

Figure 153. James Moriarty

ANSWER

Dr. Holmes interpreted the barium swallow as showing the entire length of the esophagus to be diseased. The diameter was narrowed, with an irregular contour to the margins. Fluoroscopic examination showed decreased distensibility of the esophagus and normal peristaltic waves that were dampened in amplitude. Dr. Holmes interpreted the changes as indicative of a long esophageal stricture and questioned Mrs. Moriarty about her recent household chores. Apparently, about three weeks before *James* was admitted to the hospital, his mother had been cleaning her stove. There was a small amount of the cleaning agent left in the can when she threw it onto the trash pile in the backyard. A few hours later, the child came running indoors complaining of severe burning in his mouth. The next day, he was taken to the doctor and the diagnosis of aphthous stomatitis was made.

The radiographs on the opposite page demonstrate the late changes of a "lye burn" of the esophagus. The cleansing products used for cleaning stoves contain a high percentage of sodium and potassium hydroxide. Usually, burns are seen in the mouth unless the child spits the substance out immediately. No damage is done in the stomach because the alkali is neutralized by hydrochloric acid. In the esophagus, lye is in contact with the walls for a long enough time to allow superficial and deep burns to develop. These heal with stricture formation, which is what we see here.

Treatment begins with prevention—keeping such material away from children. After the damage is done, steroid therapy may be used to reduce the inflammation. After strictures have formed, esophageal dilation with bougies is necessary. If that fails, it is sometimes necessary to interpose a segment of the colon between the cervical esophagus and the stomach.

Currently, *James* is undergoing a trial of esophageal dilation with bougies of gradually increasing size. He has continued difficulty with swallowing, and it is thought that he will never have normal pharyngeal and esophageal function again.

It's no doubt clear to everyone by now that the names have been changed to protect the innocent. In this part of the abdominal section, all the names come from the characters in the Sherlock Holmes stories.

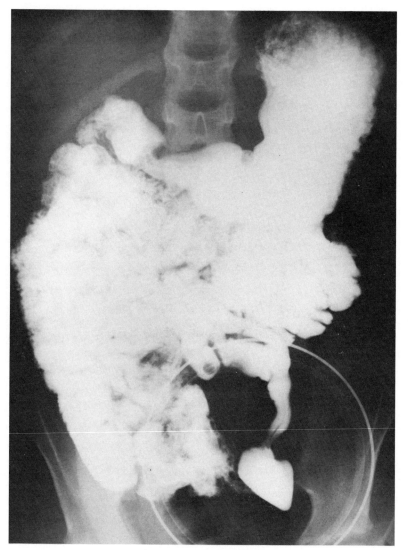

Figure 154. Daulat Ras

Daulat Ras is being evaluated because of painless rectal bleeding.

ANSWER

This radiograph obtained during *Daulat Ras'* small bowel series shows a diverticulum near the distal ileum. Do you know the eponym for this lesion? If you answered Meckel's diverticulum, you are indeed correct!

A Meckel's diverticulum is a partial remnant of the embryonic vitelline duct. It usually causes no symptoms, but occasionally it is responsible for intestinal hemorrhage or obstruction. When hemorrhage occurs, it is usually the result of ulcerations caused by the acid production of ectopic gastric mucosa in the Meckel's diverticulum. In fact, the most common cause of rectal bleeding at age 2 years is this lesion. The most sensitive way to detect a bleeding Meckel's diverticulum is not by doing barium examinations of the intestines but by performing a radionuclide scan with technetium pertechnetate (Fig. 155). If ectopic gastric mucosa is present in the diverticulum, it secretes the labelled pertechnetate and becomes a "hot spot" on the scan (arrow). Keep in mind, though, that this study does have a relatively high false-negative rate.

Why does Meckel's diverticulum cause obstruction? There are two mechanisms: intussusception of the diverticulum, and volvulus about a fibrous cord remnant of the vitelline duct. In any event, surgery is required to prevent the continued complications of this congenital lesion.

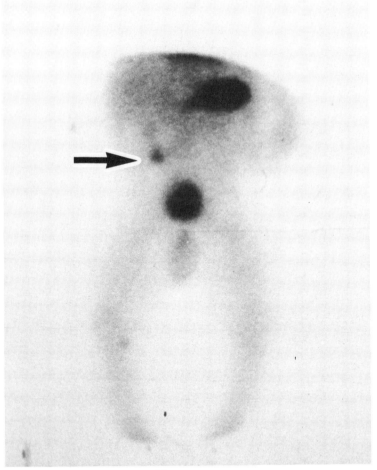

Figure 155.

FOUR CHILDREN WITH BED-WETTING

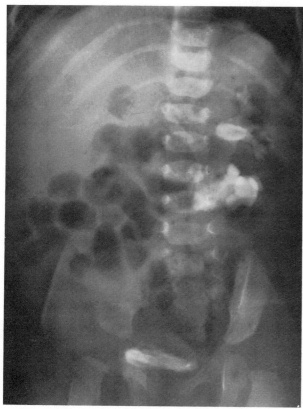

Figure 156. Charley Once-a-Week

Below and on the opposite page are excretory urograms on four children with bed-wetting problems. Their physical examinations are normal, as are their urinalyses. The parents are upset and want the radiologist to find an organic cause for the bed-wetting that can be cured easily and quickly.

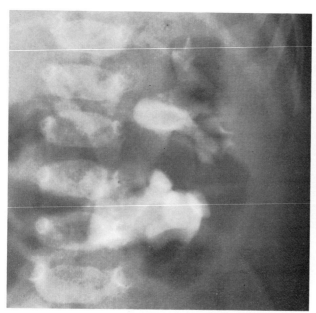

Figure 157. Charley Once-a-Week

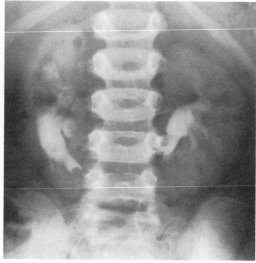

Figure 158. Harry Twice-a-Week

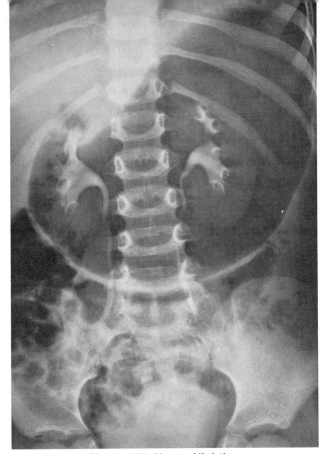

Figure 159. Nancy Nightly

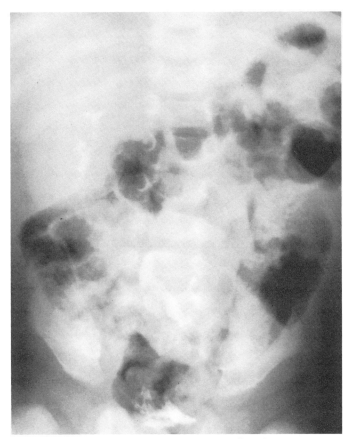

Figure 160. Earl Everyday-but-Sunday

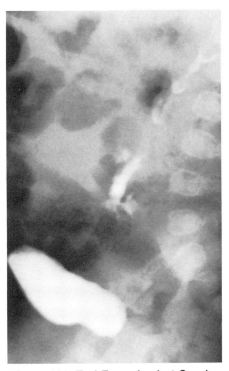

Figure 161. Earl Everyday-but-Sunday

ANSWERS

Charley Once-a-Week's excretory urogram shows two sets of opacified collecting systems on the same side of the spine. No kidney tissue is seen in the right side of the abdomen or in the pelvis. The upper set of calyces appears reasonably normal, but the lower set appears peculiar. Other films showed that the ureters enter the bladder normally.

This is crossed renal ectopia. An ectopic kidney is one that has never reached its normal position. Ectopic kidneys may be fused or nonfused to their mates, and their blood supply may be normal or anomalous. There is an increased incidence of both renal calculi and urinary tract infections in this condition. *Charley Once-a-Week's* parents were disappointed to learn that crossed renal ectopia, by itself, is not the cause of *Charley's* bed-wetting. The slight dilatation of the lower pelvis is common and perhaps normal in this condition.

Harry Twice-a-Week's kidneys are fused at their lower poles. The calyces of the right kidney are directed posteriorly and slightly medially, and the right ureter can be seen to be passing laterally. There is probably fusion of renal tissue at the inferior pole of the kidneys, but sometimes in this condition only fibrous fusion occurs. The ureters course anteriorly over the fused segment.

Harry has a horseshoe kidney. As in crossed renal ectopia, calculi and infection may be associated with this anomaly. Horseshoe kidney by itself is not a direct cause of bed-wetting, however.

Nancy Nightly, a 6 year old girl, has an entirely normal excretory urogram. The stomach has been distended by giving *Nancy* a carbonated beverage. This distention of the stomach has displaced the small bowel and allowed excellent visualization of the kidneys.

Earl Everyday-but-Sunday has a pelvic kidney, that is, a kidney located within or just above the bony pelvis.

Both *Earl* and *Charley* were firstborns. Their parents were unaware that bladder control cannot be expected in a child under the age of 2 years. (Did you notice that *Earl's* and *Charley's* capital femoral epiphyses have not yet appeared? Both children are less than 1 year old.)

As for *Nancy* and *Harry*, the cause of their bed-wetting remains unknown. Various organic abnormalities, including spina bifida occulta, and various psychiatric theories have been proposed to explain bed-wetting. Numerous treatments and medications have come into vogue and then faded away. It seems then that usually the cause of bed-wetting is unknown, but certainly there is often a large emotional component to this disorder.

FIVE MORE PATIENTS WITH ABNORMALITIES OF THE URINARY SYSTEM

Baby Boy Geldwasser, 2 days old, had passed only a few drops of urine since birth. The baby did not appear ill, but both kidneys and the bladder were easily palpable. He was referred for a *voiding cystourethrogram.* In performing a "VCUG," a sterile catheter is passed into the bladder and water-soluble contrast material is instilled. As soon as the baby starts to void around the catheter, the catheter is removed and spot films are taken.

Figure 162 demonstrates the narrow caliber of the anterior urethra. The more proximal urethra, the prostatic urethra, is markedly dilated. At the junction of the two segments of urethra are very thin folds of uroepithelium. Usually the folds cannot be seen on the VCUG, but the severe obstruction caused by these posterior urethral valves can be seen. They cause the abrupt change in the caliber of the urethra, well shown in Figure 162. The valves resemble the cusps of the aortic valve in that upon micturition they balloon *outward,* much as the aortic valve leaflets balloon *inward* during diastole. The posterior urethral valves form an obstruction that leads to bladder distention, diverticulum formation, bilateral ureteral reflux, and bilateral hydronephrosis. Figure 162 demonstrates a bladder diverticulum displacing one ureter posteriorly, and Figure 163 shows the striking hydroureter and left hydronephrosis. Further films showed the hydronephrosis to be bilateral.

Initial treatment consists of relieving the obstruction either by a diversion procedure, such as bilateral nephrostomy or ureterostomy, or by resection of the valves.

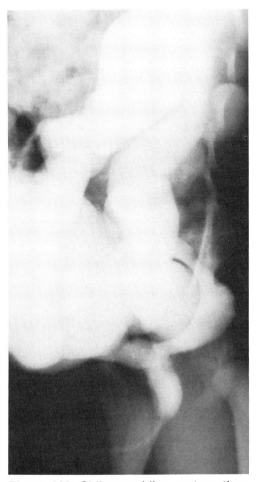

Figure 162. Oblique voiding cystourethrogram

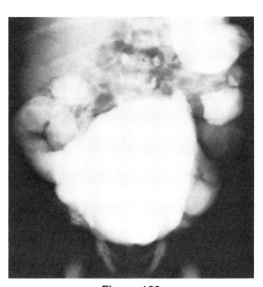

Figure 163.

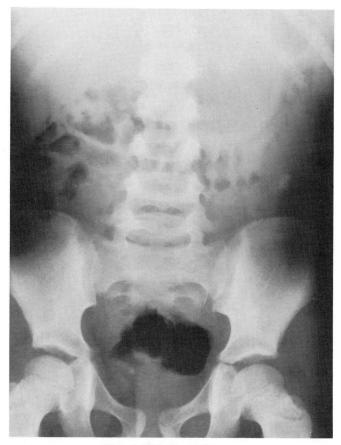

Figure 164. Stone Henge

Stone Henge, a 6 year old boy, was sent from the Emergency Room to the Radiology Department for an IVP. His mother had brought *Stone* to the hospital because of vomiting, pain in the lower abdomen radiating to the right testicle, and frequent urination. This was the first such attack.

The physical examination was difficult because the child was in considerable pain and was unable to cooperate. The urinalysis demonstrated WBCs TNTC (too numerous to count) and scattered bacteria.

Pictured here is the preliminary radiograph taken prior to injection of IVP contrast material (Fig. 164).

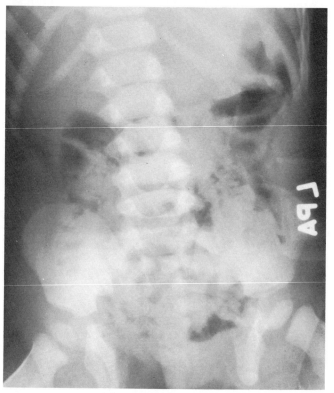

Figure 165. Bobby X.

When **Bobby X.** was born, it was obvious that he had a major abnormality in his genitourinary system. His bladder opened directly onto the lower abdominal wall. The trigone of the bladder as well as both ureteral openings were clearly visible, and the urine spilled out onto the anterior abdominal wall. The penis was foreshortened, and epispadias was evident. Figure 165 shows the preliminary view for an IVP.

Phil Hydron, a 6 month old boy, was seen because of a mass in the left upper quadrant of the abdomen. This radiograph (Fig. 166) was obtained five minutes after injection of urographic contrast material. Why is the stomach so distended?

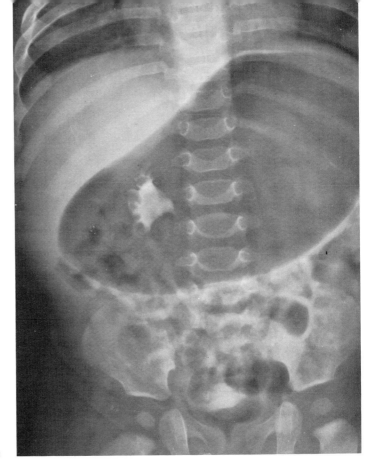

Figure 166. Phil Hydron

Ronald Reflux, age 5, has had urinary tract infections much of his life. His x-ray workup has included repeated voiding cystourethrograms and IVPs. Unfortunately, the chart, the radiographs, and the reports are unavailable at the time this IVP is "set up" for interpretation. Should you read the films or put them aside until the previous studies are available? The left kidney appears shrunken, and the calyces are clubbed. Is it enough simply to report the various causes for this radiographic appearance?

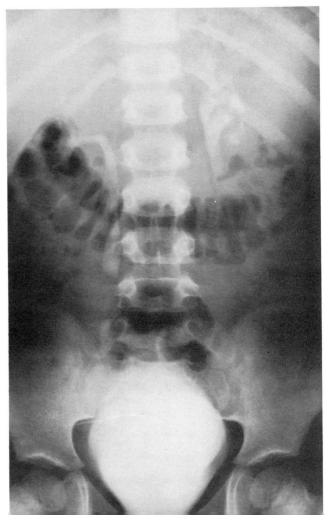

Figure 167. Ronald Reflux

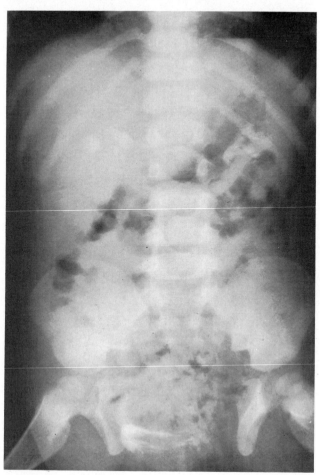

Figure 168. Stone Henge

Figure 169. Bobby X.

ANSWERS

Stone's preliminary radiograph suggested that a calculus might be present at the right ureterovesical junction. Figure 168 is a delayed radiograph from his IVP (the contrast material has already been propelled out of the left kidney), and it shows distended calyces in the right kidney and opacification of the entire course of the right ureter. The obstruction is incomplete and acute because the excretory function of the right kidney is well preserved. In total acute obstruction there may be little or no detectable urographic function of the affected kidney.

Stone passed the calculus spontaneously. He was treated for his urinary tract infection and was evaluated to determine if a cause for the calculus formation could be established. There was no evidence of cystinuria, vitamin D intoxication, hyperparathyroidism, renal tubular acidosis, or sulfonamide therapy. He has not had another urinary tract infection, nor has he formed another stone, and the explanation for the formation of this calculus remains unknown.

Bobby X.'s physical findings established the diagnosis of exstrophy of the bladder. Always associated with this anomaly is diastasis of the symphysis pubis (separation and rotation of the pubic bones). The contrast material is spilling out of the bladder onto the abdominal wall. The left kidney is small and has calyces that are crowded together and malformed. These changes were secondary to repeated urinary tract infections.

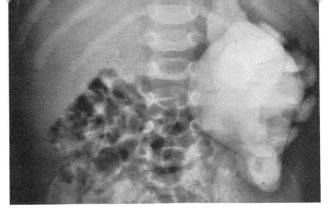

Figure 170. Phil Hydron

Phil's initial radiograph obtained five minutes after contrast material was injected gave insufficient information about the left kidney. A delayed radiograph (seven hours, Fig. 170) shows striking hydronephrosis of the left kidney. This would have been less apparent if the study had been terminated earlier, and demonstrates the value of the delayed radiograph in obstructive uropathy.

Why is the stomach distended with gas on the first radiograph? Because the child was fed a carbonated beverage—but we have been through that already.

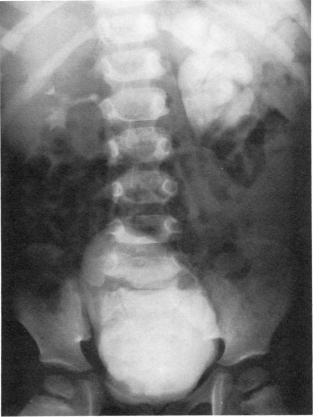

Figure 171. Ronald Reflux

Fortunately, you decided not to read *Ronald's* current IVP until you had previous films for comparison. An earlier IVP (Fig. 171) showed striking dilatation of the calyces of the left kidney. Figure 172 is a "spot film" from a VCUG. (Can you see the catheter in the urethra?) It shows reflux from the bladder into the left ureter.

The role of vesicoureteral reflux in causing renal atrophy and the place of infections in causing reflux (or is it the reflux that allows the infection?) are highly controversial. *Ronald* had both urinary tract infections and vesicoureteral reflux, and his left kidney was small and scarred. In many cases this can be prevented by long-term antibiotic therapy for the infections. Surgery may be needed to reimplant the ureter and prevent further reflux.

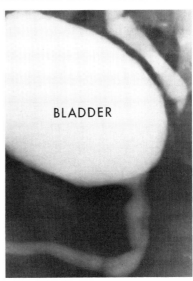

Figure 172. Ronald Reflux

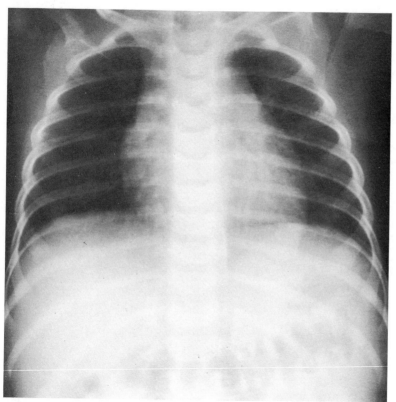

Figure 173. S. Lyme

This chest radiograph on **Spencer Lyme** was obtained because of symptoms of an upper respiratory tract infection.

ANSWER

Guess what! The focus of this case is not the chest; it is normal. What else do you see?

Observe that there are symmetrical, roughly triangular-shaped areas of calcification in the paraspinal regions of the upper abdomen. What is the organ that lives here? The adrenal glands, of course!

Bilateral calcification of normal-sized adrenal glands is often seen as an incidental finding. It is thought that this calcification is caused by clinically silent neonatal hemorrhage. Another cause of bilateral adrenal calcification is the rare condition known as Wolman disease (primary familial xanthomatosis). In this condition the patient is ill with vomiting, diarrhea, and hepatosplenomegaly, and the adrenal glands are markedly enlarged.

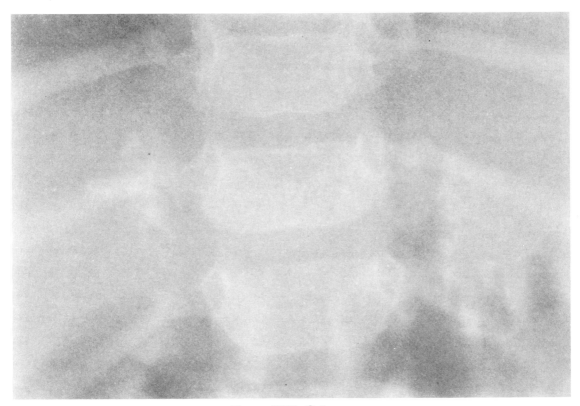

Figure 173A. S. Lyme

A LARGE MASS ON THE BACK OF A NEWBORN

Mrs. Tulp, a 28 year old woman, had been in labor for 22 hours without making progress. The baby began to show signs of fetal distress, which necessitated a cesarean section. The cause for the arrest of labor was found to be a large mass on the back of the baby in the midline, extending from the lower thoracic region to just above the buttocks. Radiographs of the mass, which was protected by a bandage, were obtained, as well as skull films. Why were the skull films obtained? What is the diagnosis, and what other diagnoses can you establish?

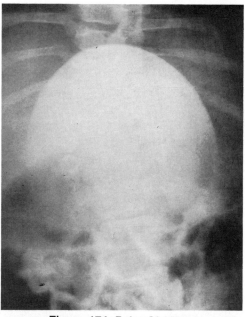
Figure 174. Baby Girl Tulp

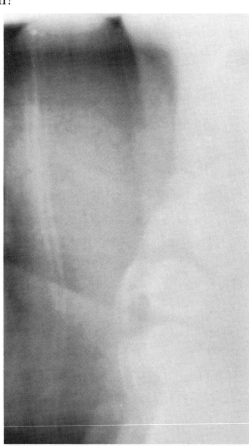
Figure 175. Baby Girl Tulp

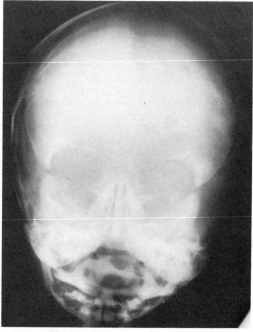
Figure 176. Baby Girl Tulp

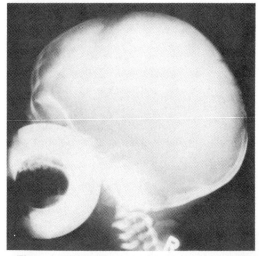
Figure 177. Baby Girl Tulp

ANSWER

Baby Girl Tulp's large mass is well seen in Figure 174 because, being outside the body, it is outlined by air. Look through the mass at the spine. The pedicles are splayed throughout the lumbar region. The extent of the osseous defect is better seen later after the mass had been removed (Fig. 178). The splayed pedicles are seen to extend throughout the lumbar and sacral regions. The change in the appearance of the pedicles is accompanied by widening of the interpediculate distance. *Baby Girl Tulp* has a meningocele; however, if nerve roots or spinal cord are included within the mass, the condition is known as a meningomyelocele.

There was gross neurologic deficit inferior to the mass. The baby dribbled urine occasionally, but no vigorous stream was ever observed. An IVP performed when the baby was older (Fig. 179) showed multiple diverticula protruding from an elongated bladder. This is the appearance of a neurogenic bladder (Fig. 180).

The radiopaque marker seen over the right acetabulum (Fig. 179) is the tip of a ventriculoperitoneal shunt catheter. A very common finding associated with meningomyelocele is hydrocephalus and Arnold-Chiari malformation. Aqueductal stenosis may also occur with meningocele. These obstructive conditions are treated by diversion procedures such as a ventriculoperitoneal shunt.

The skull radiographs demonstrate thinning of the calvaria; this is especially well seen in the frontal region. The skull has been termed "lacuna skull," or lückenschädel. It is seen almost exclusively in association with meningomyelocele or encephalocele. The local thinning of lacunar skull is much more pronounced than the convolutional markings seen normally.

(Of course you recognize the doughnut-shaped structure seen on the lateral skull radiograph as a roll of adhesive tape!)

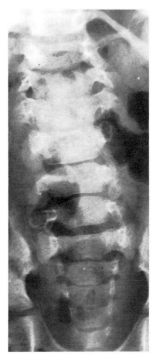

Figure 178. Baby Girl Tulp

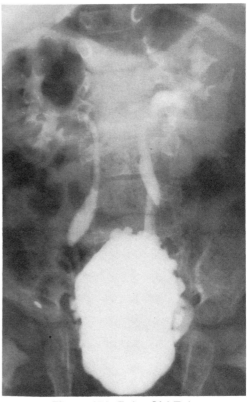

Figure 179. Baby Girl Tulp

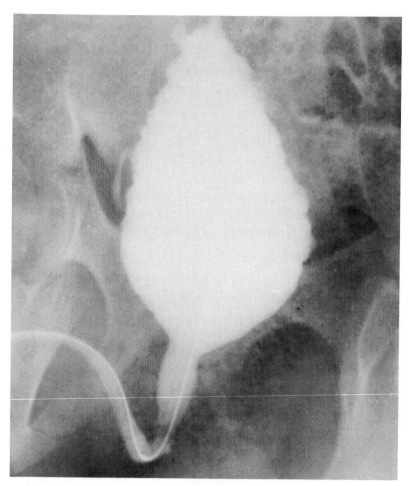

Figure 180.

Figure 180 illustrates a common appearance of a neurogenic bladder. Some investigators liken the shape of the neurogenic bladder to a Christmas tree. Multiple trabeculations and diverticula are seen as the mucosa protrudes between muscular fibers. In this case, right-sided vesicoureteral reflux is also present. Another common finding in children with a neurogenic bladder is a relaxed, patulous, and dilated bladder neck, which is illustrated here.

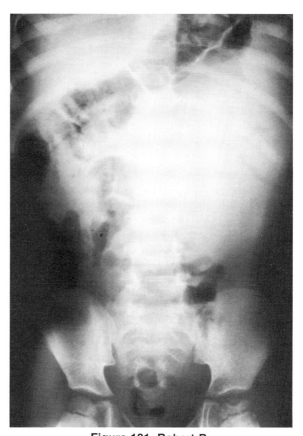

Figure 181. Robert B.

Robert Baleun is a 5 year old boy who was evaluated because of "trouble with urination for his entire life." The excretory urogram illustrated here was performed to gain anatomic information about the urinary system and to assess a mass that was palpated on the left side of the abdomen. What are the conclusions that you can reach from this study?

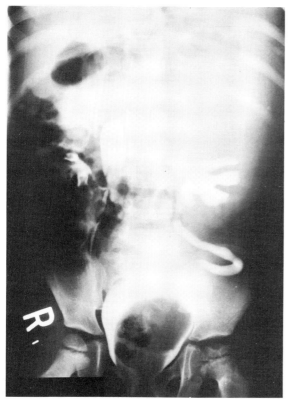

Figure 182. Robert B.

ANSWER

The abdominal scout radiograph (Fig. 181) confirms the presence of a large left-sided abdominal mass that displaces loops of gut toward the right. The second radiograph, obtained after intravenous injection of contrast material, shows that there are bilateral duplication anomalies of the collecting systems of the kidneys. Now pay attention to the left kidney. The mass that was palpated and that displaced the loops of the gut is an obstructed, hydronephrotic, upper pole collecting system of the duplicated left kidney. Why is obstruction present? The answer is submerged in a sea of urine in the bladder.

As you look at the bladder, we hope that the first thing that impresses you is the huge, round, radiolucent filling defect. This is called an ectopic ureterocele and represents the very dilated distal portion of the left upper pole ureter. This upper pole moiety ureter inserts into the bladder in a more medial and inferior position than is normal. In doing so, it has traversed the sphincter of the bladder, and the muscular contraction of the bladder sphincter has caused chronic obstruction. Why then does a portion of the ureter herniate into the lumen of the bladder? As the ureter tunnels through the submucosal region of the bladder wall, it is supported exteriorly by bladder musculature but interiorly by the weaker bladder mucosa, which is not strong enough to prevent the ureter from ballooning into the bladder.

Although the ureter of the upper pole system of a duplication anomaly is often affected by obstruction, the ureter from the lower pole moiety is often found to show vesicoureteral reflux on voiding cystourethrography. This results from abnormal intravesical wall tunneling of this ureter, which inserts into the normal trigonal position. (By the way, did you notice the abnormal ossification of the left capital femoral epiphysis?)

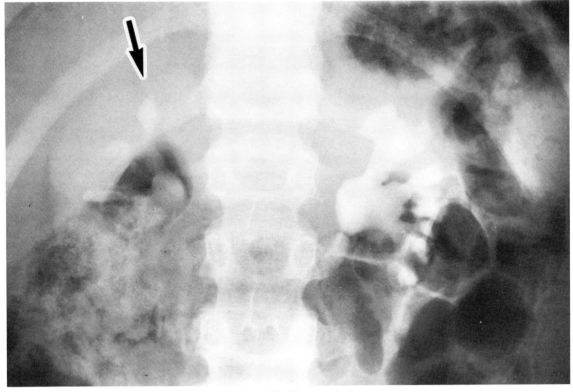

Figure 183. Margaret K.

Margaret Kramer is a 3 year old girl with a life-long history of recurrent urinary tract infections. Illustrated here is a radiograph of the kidneys obtained as part of an excretory urogram. Look at the cortex of the right kidney. What is your diagnosis?

ANSWER

The lobulated contour to the cortex of the right kidney accompanied by areas of cortical thinning adjacent to blunted calyces (arrow) indicates that *Margaret* has chronic pyelonephritis. The repeated infections have caused renal cortical and medullary tissue to become replaced by scar formation with a reduction in distance between the outer edge of the kidney and the calyces, resulting in the lobulated appearance of the kidney's contour. The right kidney demonstrates the classic radiographic findings of chronic pyelonephritis.

TWO CHILDREN WITH ABDOMINAL MASSES . . .

The following two cases involve children who had excretory urograms performed because of an abdominal mass.

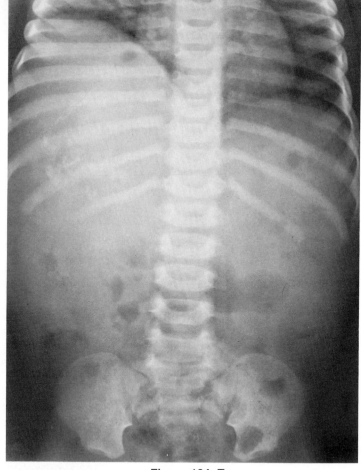

Figure 184. Tom

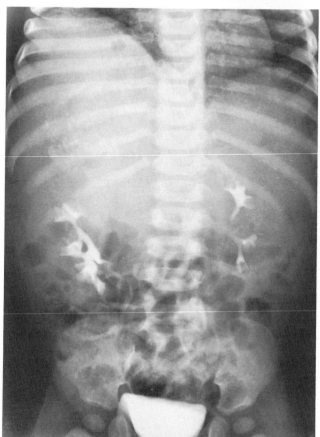

Tom, a 1½ year old boy, had fever, weight loss, and diarrhea lasting four months. Physical examination suggested consolidation in the right lower lobe of the lung. An abdominal film showed a large mass in the right upper quadrant, which contained calcifications. An IVP was performed, and the relationship of the mass to the kidney suggested the diagnosis. Can you decide what it was?

Figure 185. Tom

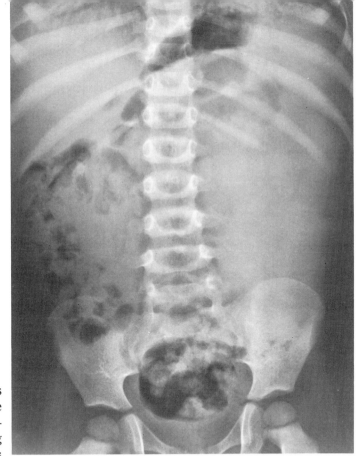

Figure 186. Ellen

Ellen, a 7 month old girl, was brought to the hospital because her mother had noticed an abdominal mass while bathing her. She claimed that the mass was not present the previous day. Bleeding into a mass may cause sudden increase in size, making it palpable. After the IVP was studied, a provisional diagnosis and treatment plan were established. How would you interpret the study?

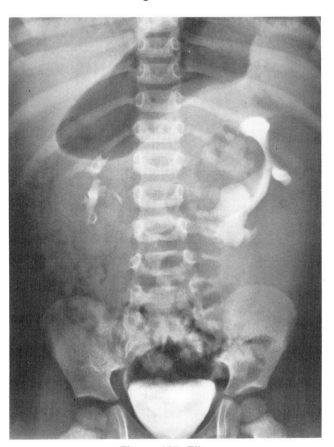

Figure 187. Ellen

ANSWERS

Tom's preliminary film shows amorphous calcification in the right upper quadrant of the abdomen. The mass has elevated the right hemidiaphragm. The excretory urogram demonstrates that the internal architecture of the right kidney is normal, but the axis of the kidney has been altered and displaced inferiorly. These findings indicate that the mass is *extrinsic* to the kidney. The calcification seen here is common in neuroblastoma.

Neuroblastomas may arise from the adrenal medulla and also from the sympathetic nervous system. Rarely, a neuroblastoma may change spontaneously to a more benign tumor. Neuroblastomas usually occur before age 4 years, with a maximal incidence at 18 months.

The frequent manifestations of neuroblastoma are abdominal mass, failure to thrive, and failure to gain weight. Many babies have metastases to the liver or bone at the time of initial examination. The laboratory evaluation includes assessment of urinary degradation products of norepinephrine, dopa, and dopamine. These substances are produced by the neuroblastoma cells and are detectable in the urine in more than nine out of ten cases. Bone marrow biopsy may disclose tumor cells in the marrow cavity long before radiographic changes are apparent.

Treatment is primarily surgical, but radiation therapy and chemotherapy have been shown to increase survival rate markedly. Prognosis is best in patients under the age of 1 year and in those without metastases. Bone involvement that is apparent radiologically indicates a poor prognosis.

Ellen has a large mass in the left upper quadrant of the abdomen. No calcification is present, and no distinguishing features are seen in the mass (except that it indents the stomach air bubble). Urographic contrast material was injected into a foot vein, and AP and lateral views of the abdomen were obtained. No compression, obstruction, or displacement of the inferior vena cava was seen. The routine IVP radiographs (Figs. 186 and 187) showed that the right kidney appeared normal but that the calyces of the left kidney were markedly distorted and separated.

These findings establish that the mass is an *intrinsic* renal mass. The most common malignant *intrinsic* renal mass of childhood is Wilms' tumor. (Yes, this is spelled correctly—the man's name was Max Wilms.)

The most common symptom is abdominal mass; however, pain and fever may occur, as well as hypertension. The association of Wilms' tumor with hemihypertrophy of both soft tissues and skeleton and aniridia (no iris) is well known but not commonly seen.

The workup may be supplemented with angiography to demonstrate the extent of the tumor and to determine if there is growth of the neoplasm into the renal vein and inferior vena cava. If this is found, measures can be taken to prevent tumor emboli from reaching the lungs. In this regard, if Wilms' tumor is suspected clinically, palpation of the abdomen should be kept to a minimum.

Treatment of Wilms' tumor is aimed at primary excision of the tumor with the capsule intact. Postoperative radiotherapy has been found to increase the number of survivors. Chemotherapy, notably actinomycin D, also increases the survival rate, and both chemotherapy and radiotherapy are used in most treatment plans currently. When metastases occur in Wilms tumor, the lungs and liver are common sites, but the bones are rarely involved.

It should be noted that the use of ultrasound, computed tomography, and magnetic resonance imaging in the differentiation and staging of abdominal masses is gradually replacing urography and angiography.

AND ANOTHER CHILD WITH AN ABDOMINAL MASS . . .

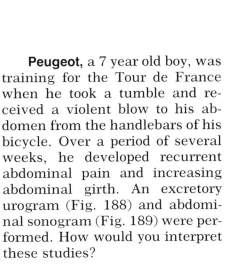

Peugeot, a 7 year old boy, was training for the Tour de France when he took a tumble and received a violent blow to his abdomen from the handlebars of his bicycle. Over a period of several weeks, he developed recurrent abdominal pain and increasing abdominal girth. An excretory urogram (Fig. 188) and abdominal sonogram (Fig. 189) were performed. How would you interpret these studies?

Figure 188. Peugeot

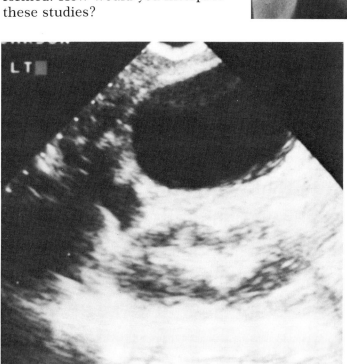

Figure 189. Peugeot

ANSWER

On the excretory urogram, we see that the left kidney is displaced inferiorly by a large soft tissue mass that lies anterior and superior to the kidney. The kidney is intrinsically normal. The sonogram is very helpful in that it shows us that the mass seen on excretory urography is in the pancreas and represents a sonolucent cyst; thus, *Peugeot* can be presumed to have a traumatic pseudocyst of the pancreas. In children, such cysts are most commonly the result of trauma, but other causes include idiopathic pancreatitis, hereditary pancreatitis, mumps, drugs (corticosteroids), and cholelithiasis.

Operative therapy is usually required for a pancreatic pseudocyst, although there are recent reports of therapeutic percutaneous transgastric drainage. Pancreatic pseudocysts may be complicated by hemorrhage; infection; peritonitis secondary to infection; and obstruction of the pancreatic ducts, biliary ducts, and gastrointestinal tracts by mass effect.

NOW YOU OUGHT TO BE READY TO INTERPRET THIS EXCRETORY UROGRAM:

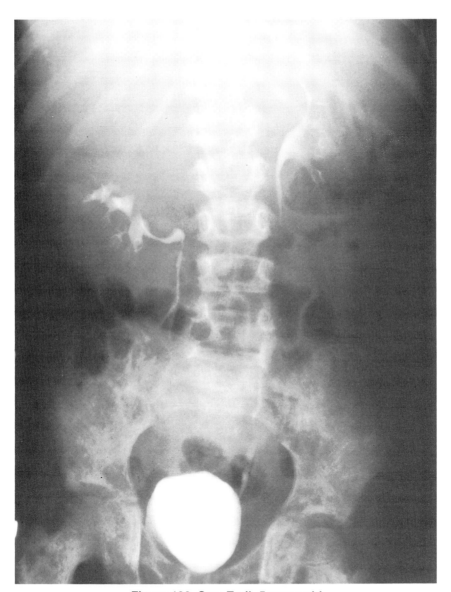

Figure 190. Sam Trail, 5 years old

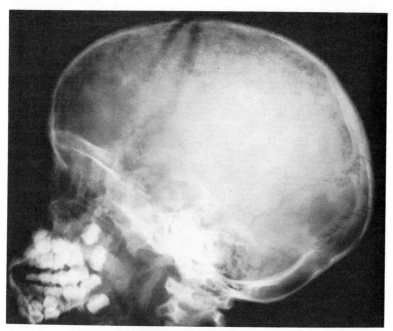

Figure 191. Sam T.

ANSWER

Sam T. was 5 years old when all radiographs shown here were obtained. AP and lateral skull films (Figs. 191 and 192) demonstrated marked diastasis of the coronal and sagittal sutures and bone destruction. These changes are caused by metastatic neuroblastoma to the dura mater and cranium.

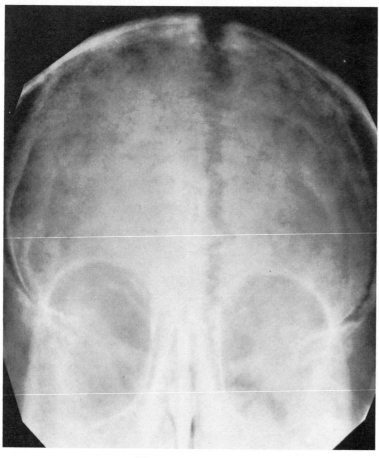

Figure 192. Sam T.

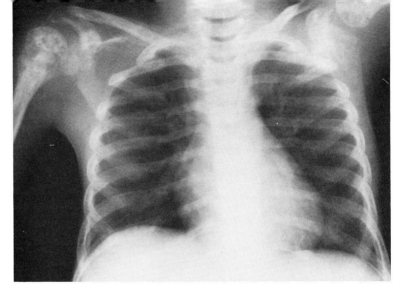

Figure 193. Sam T.

The chest radiograph (Fig. 193) demonstrates lytic changes in many of the bones. At the same time, notice that no metastatic deposits are visible in the lungs—pulmonary metastases are uncommon with neuroblastoma.

The radiographs of the arms (Fig. 194) show the symmetrical character of the metastases, one of the hallmarks of this condition. The IVP (Fig. 190) shows displacement of the right kidney from its normal axis by a mass superior to it. The calcification in the right upper quadrant was a key finding (Fig. 195, detail); together with the bone changes in the pelvis, this one film establishes that the mass is most likely a **neuroblastoma.**

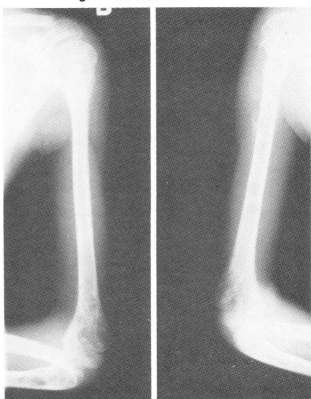

Figure 194. Sam T., right and left arms

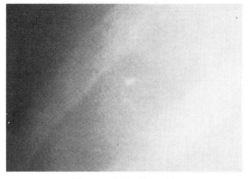

Figure 195. Sam T.

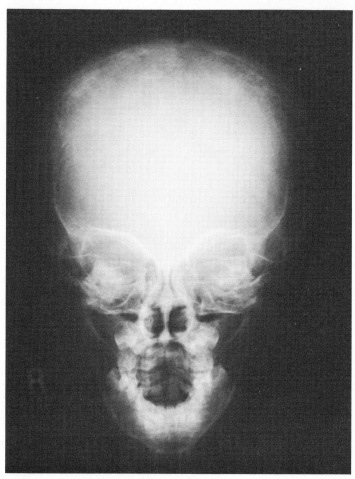

Figure 196.

Treatment for cranial metastasis from neuroblastoma results in the roentgen pattern illustrated in Figures 196 and 197. Note the cranial changes, which include foci of lucency and density and the thickening of the calvarium.

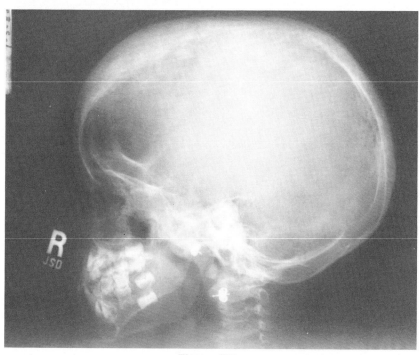

Figure 197.

HOW ABOUT ANOTHER PATIENT WITH AN ABDOMINAL MASS . . .

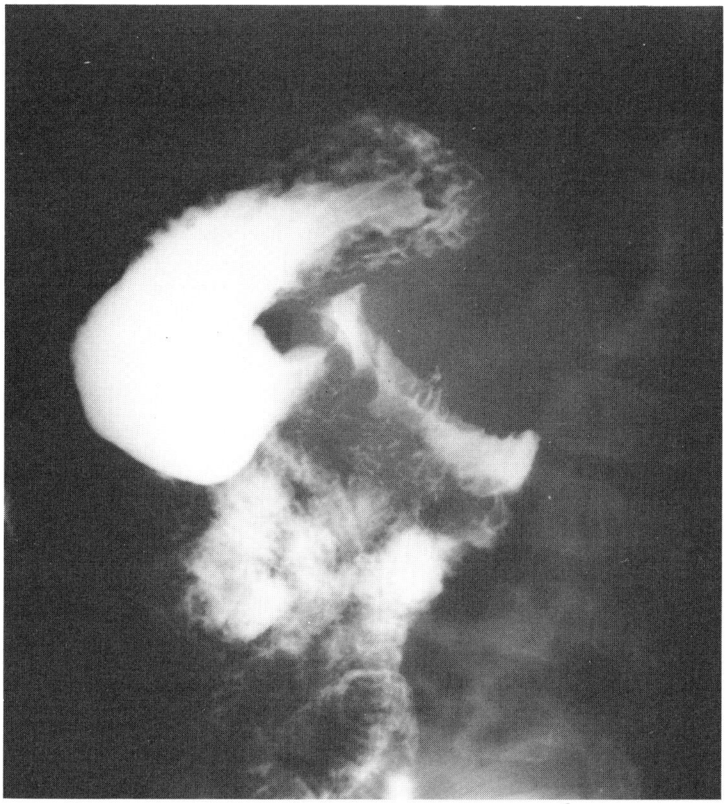

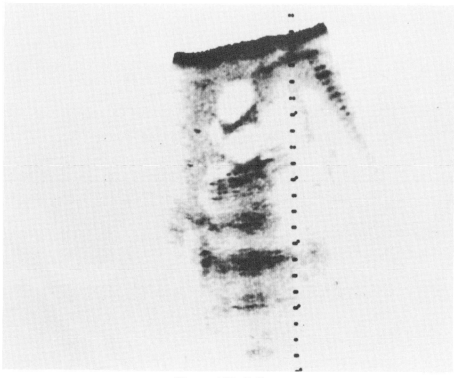

Celia, a 7 year old girl, was evaluated because of jaundice, abdominal pain, and a right upper quadrant abdominal mass. What is your first diagnostic consideration, and which imaging studies would you request?

Celia first had an upper gastrointestinal series (Fig. 198), and then an abdominal sonogram (Fig. 199). What is your diagnosis?

Figure 198. Celia

Figure 199. Celia

ANSWER

Anteromedial displacement of a smoothly compressed duodenal bulb is seen on the upper gastrointestinal study; the sonogram shows that the displacement is caused by a sonolucent, cystic mass. The most likely diagnosis is choledochal cyst, and hepatobiliary scintigraphy should confirm this. An intraoperative cholangiogram (Fig. 200) was performed in this case, and shows the biliary system, gallbladder, and choledochal cyst (arrow).

A choledochal cyst is a saccular dilation or a cystic diverticulum branching off from the common bile duct. Obstruction to normal bile flow commonly occurs, and jaundice and pain develop. The mass often becomes large enough to be readily palpable. At least three quarters of the patients with choledochal cyst are girls, and the age of presentation ranges from less than 1 year to adolescence.

The critical diagnostic pathway for choledochal cysts includes sonography and hepatobiliary scintigraphy. The treatment is surgical, and drainage can be accomplished by an anastomosis between the cyst and the duodenum or jejunum. Some surgeons favor excision of the cyst, if this is possible.

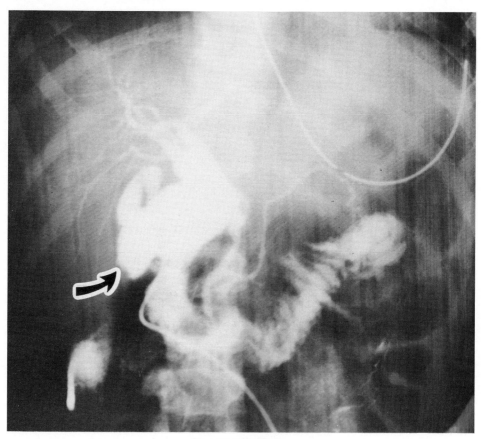

Figure 200. Celia

Skull

DIFFICULT TO CONTROL SEIZURES AND MENTAL RETARDATION

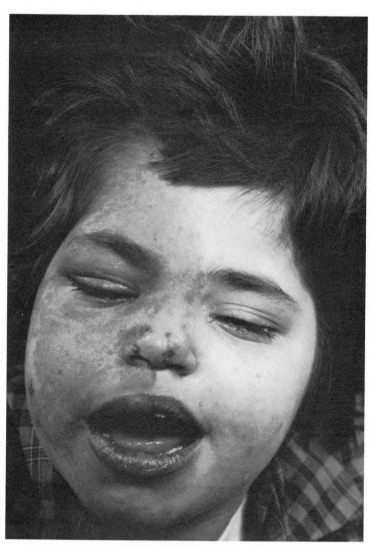

Figure 201. Mary Beth

Mary Beth (Fig. 201), age 7, had been referred to the Seizure Clinic because of increasing frequency of seizures. Her condition was recognized at birth on the basis of a purple cutaneous lesion (port-wine hemangioma) that was distributed over the area innervated by the right trigeminal nerve. *Mary Beth* was 1 year old when left-sided grand mal seizures began. Recently the seizures have occurred more frequently.

The neurologic examination demonstrated a spastic left hemiparesis and a visual field deficit. Skull radiographs confirmed the diagnosis (Figs. 202, 203, and 204).

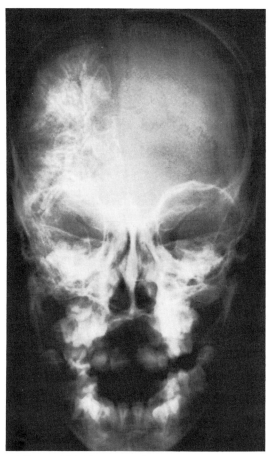

Figure 202. Frontal projection: Mary Beth

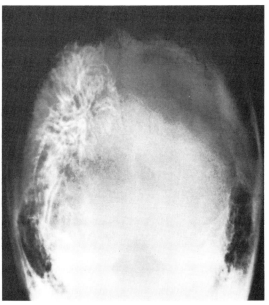

Figure 203. Towne's projection: Mary Beth

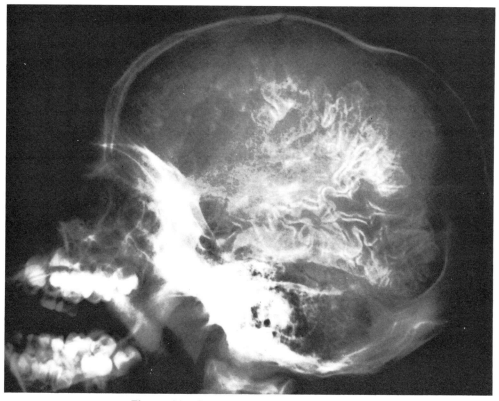

Figure 204. Lateral projection: Mary Beth

ANSWER

Mary Beth's skull radiographs demonstrate railroad track calcification extending from the occipital pole to the frontal pole of the right cerebral cortex. This is calcification of the shrunken cerebral cortical gyri. These are *not* the calcified walls of blood vessels. The port-wine hemangioma seen on the face has its counterpart in venous angiomatosis of the pia and arachnoid layers of the meninges overlying the affected area.

This is *encephalofacial angiomatosis*, or the Sturge-Weber syndrome. The affected portion of the cerebral hemisphere may be significantly smaller than its mate, resulting in failure of growth of the overlying calvaria and an asymmetrical skull.

Visual field deficit, hemiparesis, seizures, and mental retardation are clinical manifestations of the cerebral atrophy and dysfunction. Treatment is aimed at reducing the frequency of seizures with anticonvulsant medication. If the seizures are not controlled medically, surgical excision of the affected cortex may be considered.

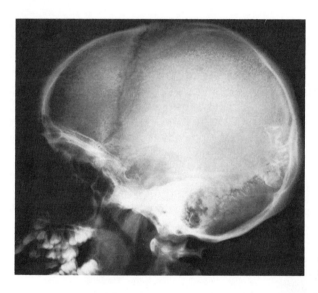

Figure 205. Another case of Sturge-Weber syndrome with less extensive calcification of the cerebral cortex

Désiré Magloire B. is a severely retarded 16 year old child with seizures and with discrete papules on the bridge of her nose and over the malar regions.

Look at her lateral skull radiograph and give us your number one diagnosis!

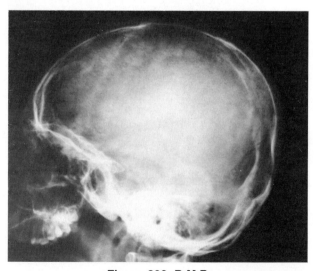

Figure 206. D.M.B.

ANSWER

The skull radiograph of *D.M.B.* shows multiple intracranial calcifications in the general distribution of the lateral ventricles. This is a common radiographic pattern for tuberous sclerosis, which is the diagnosis in this youngster. It is observed in about half the cases of tuberous sclerosis and is caused by calcifications within hamartomatous subependymal nodules. Hamartomatous tumors, usually angiomyolipomas, are also commonly found in the kidneys (Fig. 207). Note the multiple regions of neovascularity and the gross enlargement of the kidneys demonstrated on the renal arteriogram.

Other radiographic manifestations of tuberous sclerosis include sclerotic islands of bone in vertebral bodies and both sclerotic and cystic changes in the phalanges. The lungs may also be involved by interstitial fibrosis, but this is an unusual occurrence.

Tuberous sclerosis is also known by the eponym "Bourneville's disease," after the French neurologist (1840–1909) whose first name was Désiré-Magloire. This disease is characterized clinically by the classic, but certainly not always complete, triad of mental retardation, seizures, and adenoma sebaceum.

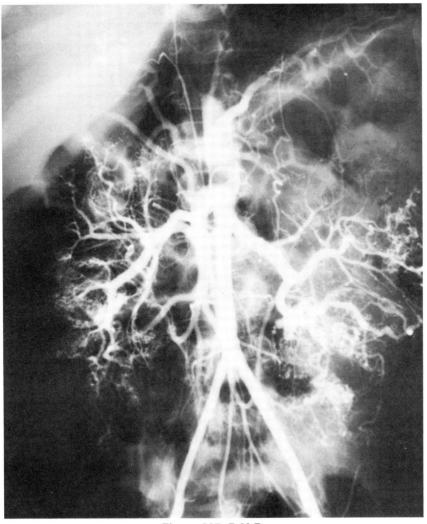

Figure 207. D.M.B.

ANOTHER PROBLEM: MULTIPLE WORMIAN BONES

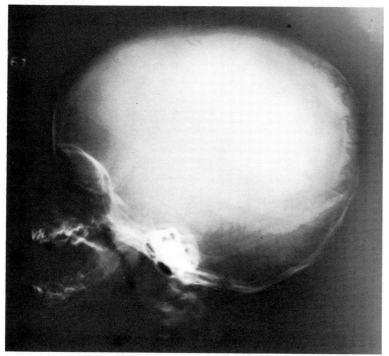

Figure 208. Frank Fragile

Notice the multiple bones in the lambdoidal suture in the patient illustrated in Figure 208, **Frank Fragile.** These bones are known as wormian bones (after the Danish anatomist Oläus Worm—not after helminths). They are areas of ossification of membranous bone that arise in the sutures and fontanelles. When there are multiple wormian bones, several conditions should come to mind. What are they?

ANSWER

Frank Fragile, a 1 year old boy, was dropped from a table, striking his head on the floor. Figures 208 and 209 show radiographs taken before and after the trauma. The first shows the wormian bones, but something has been added on the second study—multiple lucent lines. These are **skull fractures.** *Frank Fragile* has blue sclera, multiple wormian bones, and many skull and skeletal fractures. He has **osteogenesis imperfecta.**

Other conditions in which multiple wormian bones are found include cretinism, cleidocranial dysostosis, and hypophosphatasia, but normal children have them, too.

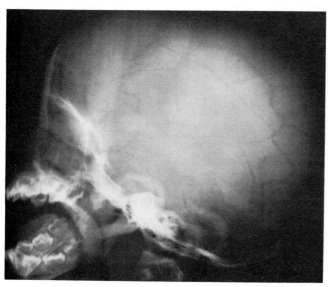

Figure 209. Frank Fragile

INTRACRANIAL CALCIFICATION

One of the common reasons pediatricians obtain skull radiographs of infants is to aid in the evaluation of slow development. **Paul C.**, a 4 year old boy, had not yet begun to talk or walk. His head was large for his body, and his forehead was especially prominent.

The radiographs suggest the cause of failure of normal growth and development. What are the special procedures that you would use to prove the *diagnosis*? (The oblique lines projected over the left orbit and across the top of the skull are artifacts. What are they?)

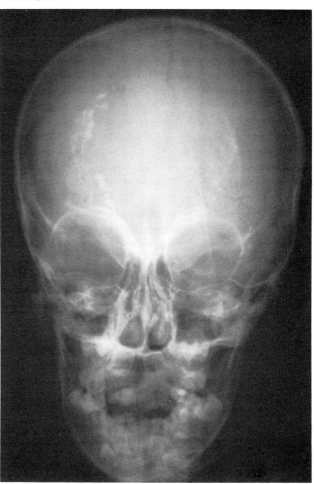

Figure 210. Paul C.

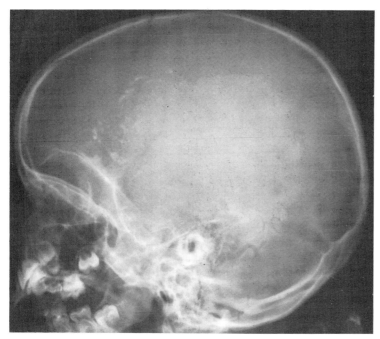

Figure 211. Paul C.

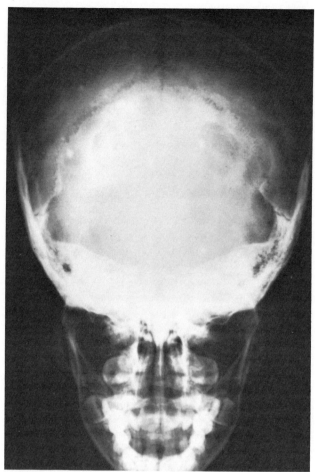

Figure 212. Harvey B.

Harvey B., a 28 month old boy, was sent by his ophthalmologist for skull radiographs because of the finding of chorioretinitis. What did the ophthalmologist think the radiographs might demonstrate?

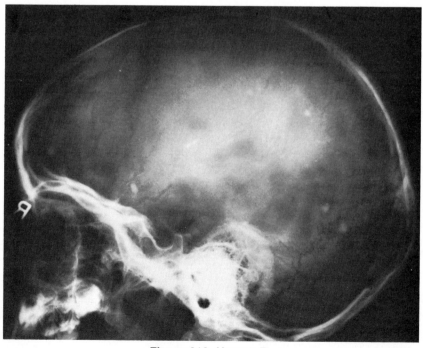

Figure 213. Harvey B.

ANSWERS

Paul C.'s skull radiographs demonstrate calcification that appears symmetrical and conforms to the expected margins of dilated lateral ventricles. In the past, the next step to test this hypothesis would be a pneumoencephalogram (Figs. 214 and 215). Today, we would use computed tomography. These radiographs confirm the location of the calcification in the walls of dilated lateral ventricles. The excessively wide sulci are outlined by air and indicate brain atrophy. *Paul* has cytomegalic inclusion disease (CID), a viral illness that may be acquired during gestation. Congenital CID infection may affect the lungs, liver, and hematopoietic system as well as the central nervous system. Unfortunately, there is no treatment for this disease.

The lines projected across *Paul's* forehead and left orbit are pieces of adhesive tape used to immobilize the patient. (An edge is seen when there is an air–adhesive tape interface.)

Harry B.'s skull radiographs show calcification distributed throughout the brain. This type and distribution of calcification are seen in another congenital infection, toxoplasmosis. *Toxoplasma* is a parasite that can sometimes be demonstrated in the cerebrospinal fluid. If the baby is not stillborn, he may be left with brain damage, microcephaly, seizures, and chorioretinitis. In this patient, the basis for the chorioretinitis was indeed toxoplasmosis.

The periventricular distribution of calcification seen in *Paul* and the diffuse distribution seen with *Harvey* are not absolutely specific for the etiologic agent. However, the calcification does indicate a congenital infection and suggests the *likely* pathogen.

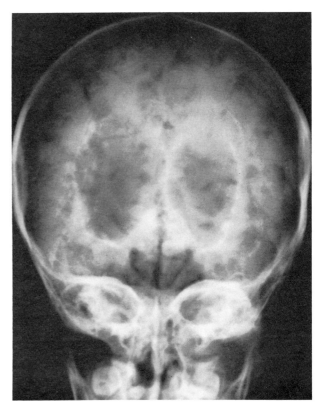

Figure 214. Paul C.

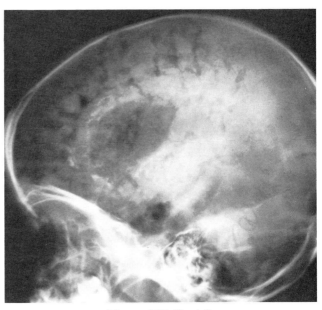

Figure 215. Paul C.

SUPRACELLAR CALCIFICATION

Karen L., a 3 year old girl, was seen initially by her pediatrician because of persistent vomiting and headache. Physical examination demonstrated papilledema, and *Karen* was admitted to the hospital, where skull radiographs were obtained. The lateral radiograph (Fig. 216) shows calcification above the sella turcica. The sella itself is enlarged, with undermining of the anterior clinoid processes and thinning of the dorsum. The coronal sutures are diastatic. What is the diagnosis?

ANSWER

Karen has a craniopharyngioma. This is a histologically benign cystic tumor that arises from epithelium that contributes to the formation of the pituitary gland. The squamous cell component of the hypophysis is slowly shed and accumulates to form a cystic mass. The expansion of this mass interrupts the flow of CSF toward the cerebral convexities, causing hydrocephalus, increased intracranial pressure, papilledema, headache, vomiting, and widened sutures. Calcification occurs in the necrotic debris of shed cells and is almost always present in children with craniopharyngioma. Visual field defects occur because of direct pressure on the optic pathways.

The aim of therapy is total excision of the craniopharyngioma. The size and location of the tumor may make this quite difficult. Furthermore, interruption of pituitary function is expected (e.g., reduced ACTH formation, diabetes insipidus). It may not be possible to remove the entire craniopharyngioma, and it is sometimes necessary to reoperate when the symptoms return.

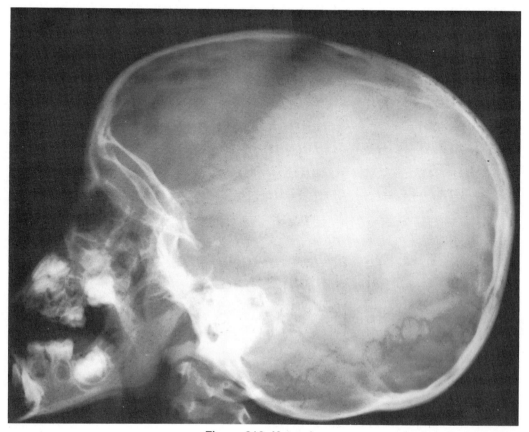

Figure 216. Karen L.

SEIZURES AND MENTAL RETARDATION (BE CAREFUL: ALL THAT GLITTERS IS NOT GOLD [OR CALCIUM])

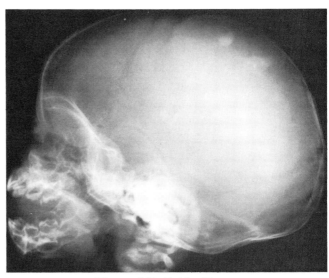

Figure 217. Bobby Bogus

Bobby Bogus, 3 years old, was clearly retarded. He also had seizures and was admitted to the hospital for manipulation of anticonvulsive drug dosage as well as for determination of the cause of the seizures and mental retardation. Included here are AP and lateral skull radiographs. What is the procedure that *Bobby* had just before the skull radiographs were taken?

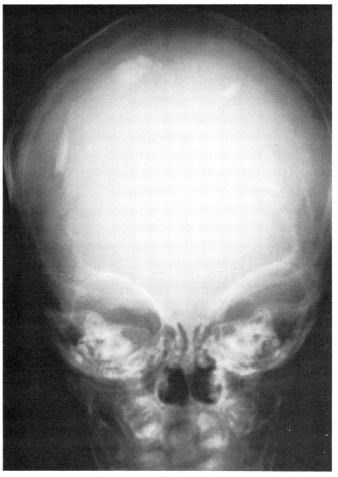

Figure 218. Bobby Bogus

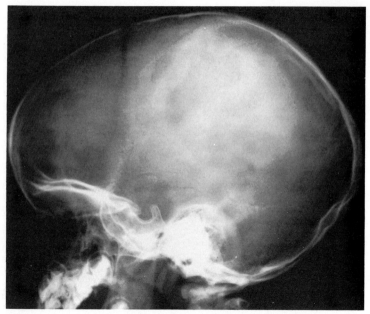

Figure 219. F. Fake

F. Fake, age 2, has the same history as *Bobby Bogus*. In this case, *F.* is a female name (*Frieda*). How can we be certain? What are the serpentine shadows projected over the parietal region on the lateral skull radiographs (Fig. 219)?

ANSWERS

At first glance, *Bobby Bogus* seems to have multiple areas of intracranial calcification. It's somewhat difficult to think of a disease that causes this pattern of calcification. In fact, *Bobby* had an electroencephalogram (EEG) just prior to coming to the Pediatric Radiology Department for his skull series. The densities seen projected over the calvaria are caused by EEG paste, which is used to ensure good conductivity between the scalp and the EEG leads. The proof is in the shampoo. After *Bobby* was shampooed, the "calcifications" disappeared. (*Bobby's* final diagnosis was idiopathic epilepsy, which has no roentgen findings.)

We can tell that *Freida Fake* is a female because of the serpentine shadows seen on the lateral skull radiographs. These are tightly wound hair braids, a style very popular with black girls.

Artifacts ("made by hand") are a very real part of radiology. It's not enough to recognize the abnormal. You must be able to separate what simulates the abnormal from what is genuinely pathologic.

TWO PATIENTS WITH UNUSUAL HEAD SHAPE

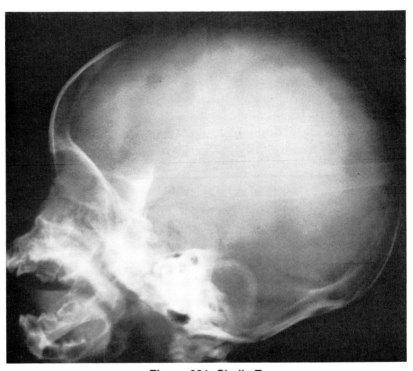

Figure 220. Sheila T.

At age 3 months, **Sheila T.** was noticed to have an asymmetrical face with a flattened left side of the forehead and orbit region. In retrospect, her parents thought that this deformity had been present since birth.

The child appeared otherwise well, and the neurologic examination was negative. These skull radiographs were obtained (Figs. 220 and 221).

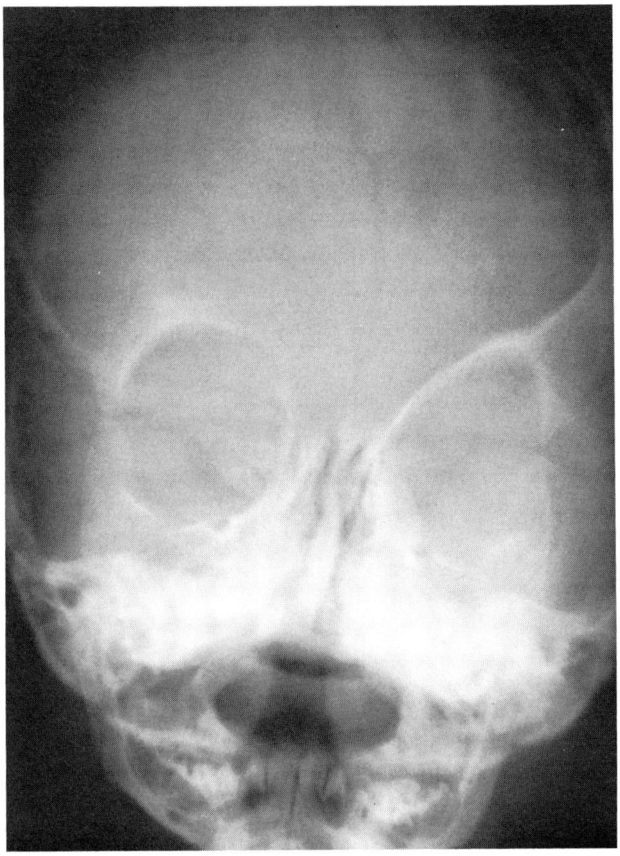

Figure 221. Sheila T.

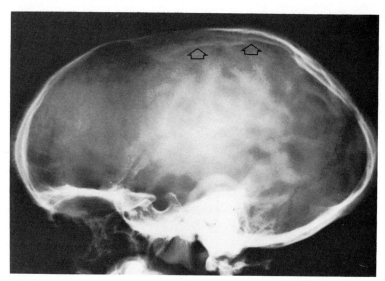

Figure 222. Harold W.

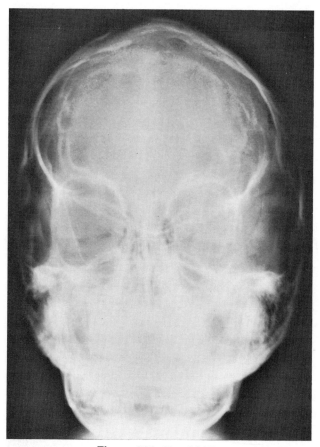

Figure 223. Harold W.

Harold W., age 5, was seen by a pediatric neurologist because of hyperactive behavior and the possibility of minimal brain damage. He had been born with a long, egg-shaped skull, but no one had thought this remarkable. These skull radiographs were obtained as part of the neurologic workup (Figs. 222, 223, and 224).

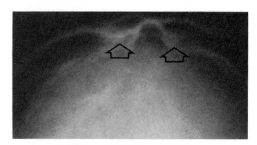

Figure 224. Harold W.

ANSWERS

Sheila T.'s orbits are asymmetrical. The right orbit is round, whereas the left orbital rim is triangular; the orbital roof is elevated and points upward and outward. The lateral view is oblique enough so that the coronal suture region on each side of the skull can be separately evaluated. No portion of the coronal suture is visible.

Sheila has premature synostosis of at least the left half of the coronal suture (judging from the orbital deformity). Because the lateral radiograph failed to demonstrate either limb of the coronal suture well, the surgeons elected to perform a bilateral excision of a strip of the calvaria in the region of the coronal sutures. To retard regrowth of bone, a polyethylene film was folded over the bone at the edges of the defect and left in place (Fig. 225).

The generic term for premature closure of the sutures is **craniosynostosis.** Normally, in a newborn baby the cranial bones are separated from each other by the sutures, which at first are merely broad strips of unossified membrane. If two or more of the calvarial bones fuse together and obliterate the suture(s) before birth or during the first few years of life, normal brain growth unduly widens those sutures that are still patent, leading to calvarial deformity. The descriptive terminology is confusing for those untutored in Greek. However, the following table lists the important and frequently used terms for the cranial malformations caused by craniosynostosis. Since the English terms describe the central pathogenetic state, whereas the Greek terms merely refer to the resulting shape, the first column probably should be used preferentially.

English	Greek	Meaning
Unilateral coronal synostosis	Plagiocephaly	Asymmetrical or twisted head
Bilateral coronal synostosis	Brachycephaly	Short head
Sagittal synostosis	Scaphocephaly	Skiff(boat)-shaped long, narrow head
Premature fusion of the sagittal and the coronal *or* ocasionally the lambdoidal sutures	Oxycephaly	Pointed head

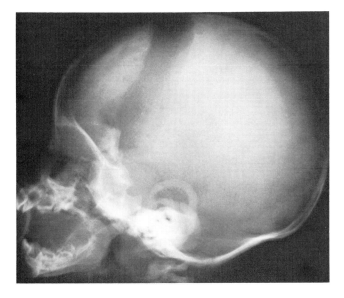

Figure 225. Sheila T.

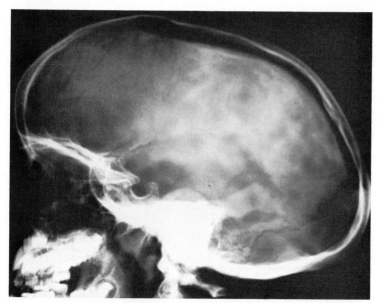

Figure 226. Harold W.

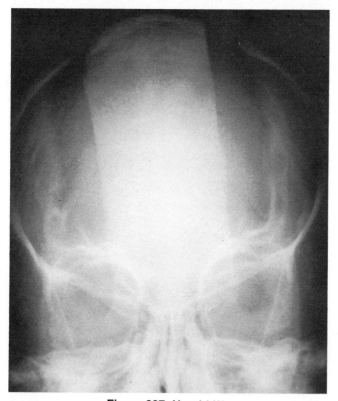

Figure 227. Harold W.

Harold W. has a markedly elongated skull with obliteration of the normal sagittal suture. The bony fusion is well seen on the coned-down (sagittal) detail view in Figure 224 (arrows). This is sagittal synostosis, or scaphocephaly, and this is the most common suture involved in craniosynostosis.

The indication for surgery in *Harold's* case was cosmetic repair of his odd skull shape, although at his age, the alteration in head shape achieved by surgery probably will be minimal. More importantly, if several sutures are involved, surgery is generally thought to be indicated for relief of restriction of brain growth, which, if untreated, would result in compression, gross distortion of the brain, probable neurologic deficit, and mental retardation. Although the extent of neurologic deficit is thought to be a function of the number of sutures involved, we have seen many children who are mentally normal despite skulls seriously deformed from premature fusion of all calvarial sutures. Possibly, brain and neurologic abnormalities in children with craniosynostosis represent associated malformations and are not the result of craniosynostosis. In *Harold's* case, sagittal synostosis alone would be unlikely to produce any neurologic impairment or mental retardation. In general, however, the greater the number of sutures that are closed, the higher the incidence of mental retardation and neurologic deficit.

Harold had a strip of bone removed from either side of the midline from just anterior to the coronal suture to just behind the lambdoidal suture (Figs. 226 and 227). A midline strip of bone was not removed because bleeding could be a problem if the sagittal sinus were inadvertently lacerated.

In *Harold's* case, the cosmetic results were not as striking as might have been expected had he been operated upon during the first year of life.

Sheila T., on the other hand, appears somewhat improved clinically, whereas if left untreated, her condition would have worsened.

HOLES IN THE HEAD

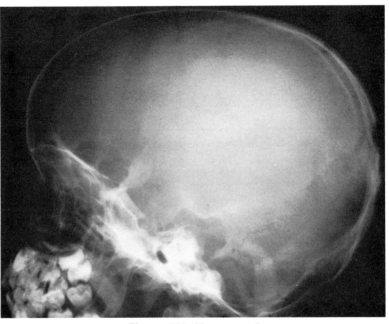

Hans S. was 2 years old when this set of skull radiographs was obtained (Figs. 228 and 229). He was irritable and seemed to have pain on palpation of his head. This was not unexpected. Approximately 1 year earlier, when the boy had a chronically draining left ear accompanied by a skin eruption that resembled seborrheic dermatitis, radiographs of the skull and of the mastoid region were obtained (Fig. 230).

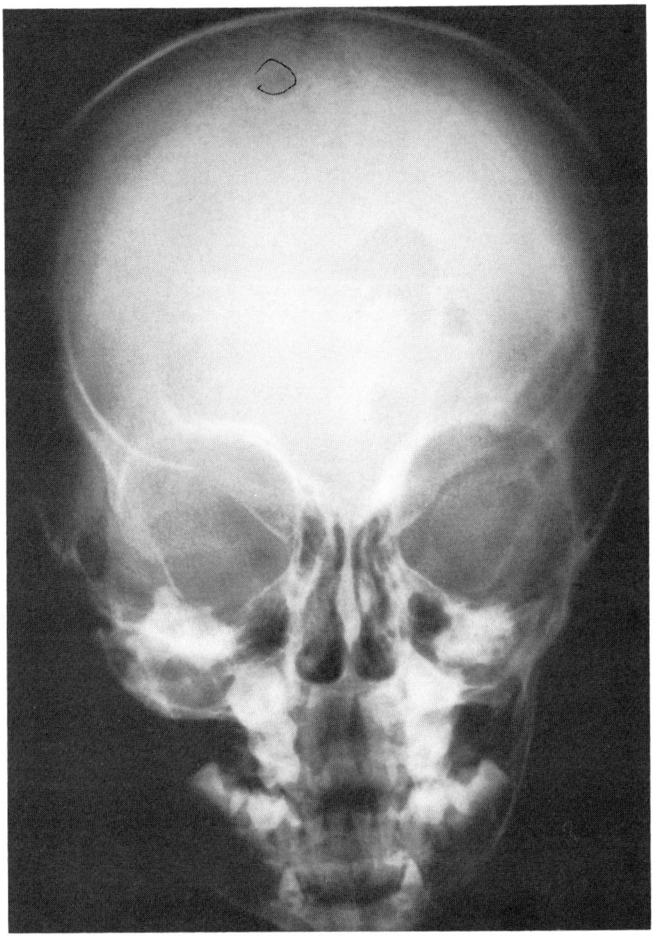

Figure 228. Hans, age 2

Figure 229. Hans, age 2

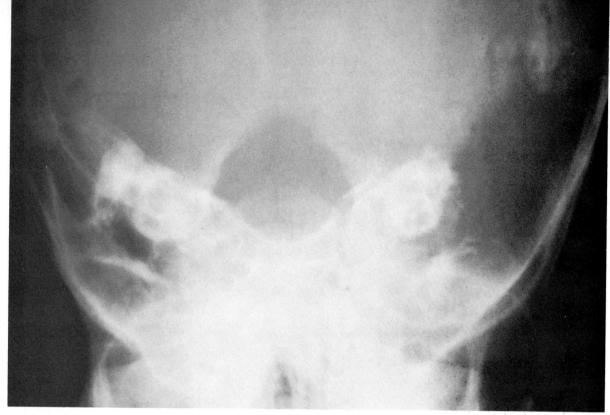

Figure 230. Hans, age 1

The diagnosis was made by biopsy of one of the skull lesions, and treatment was initiated. At age 3, however, *Hans* developed loose deciduous molars on the left side of the mandible. Radiographs shown in Figures 231 and 232 were obtained. (Figure 231 is the right side of the mandible and is the control.)

What is the diagnosis?

Figure 230 is the Towne's view of the skull. The hole in the center is the foramen magnum. Seen through it is the incompletely fused arch of the first cervical vertebra. On either side of the foramen magnum are the petrous pyramids. Are they both abnormal? These oblique views (Figs. 231 and 232) of the mandible were obtained so that each side of the mandible could be studied separately. A true lateral view of the mandible would superimpose the right and left sides, and the overlap would make interpretation difficult.

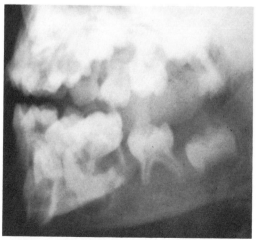

Figure 231. Hans, age 3

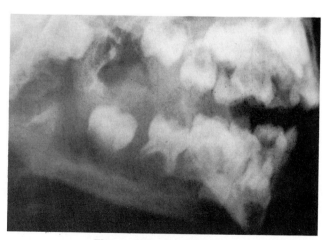

Figure 232. Hans, age 3

ANSWER

Hans S. was originally evaluated because of what was thought to be seborrheic dermatitis and left otitis media. This is not an uncommon manner of presentation for this condition.

The skull radiographs at that time showed a single punched-out lesion of bone with a smooth border. This was biopsied, and the specimen showed histiocytes, reticulum cells, and eosinophils. This was thought to represent histiocytosis X.

The Towne's view shows extensive destruction of the left mastoid. Treatment consisted of radiation therapy to the involved area and then chemotherapy. However, at age 3, *Hans* complained of loose teeth on the left side of the mandible. The radiograph (Fig. 232) of the affected area demonstrates the "floating teeth sign," which occurs when there is extensive bone destruction and the teeth are no longer firmly rooted.

Hans has extensive osseous involvement of the skull as well as involvement of the viscera. There is no evidence of pulmonary involvement yet, but *Hans* has anemia, lymph node enlargement, and hepatosplenomegaly. The lytic lesions in the skull (Figs. 228 and 229) are obvious, but did you notice the destruction of the posterior wall of the left orbit? Exophthalmos is beginning to develop.

Histiocytosis X is the generic name for three conditions previously thought to be distinct diseases. Now many authorities consider them to represent different manifestations of the same disease.

Eosinophilic granuloma has the best prognosis of these three conditions. It usually is a disease restricted to one or a few bones. Hand-Schüller-Christian disease may be manifested by (1) unilateral exophthalmos, (2) diabetes insipidus, and (3) skeletal lesions. This triad appears more commonly on board examinations than it does clinically and is worth memorizing *only* for that reason. But this is what Hans has.

The least favorable outcome occurs in the Letterer-Siwe condition. This phase of histiocytosis X may be rapidly fatal. Its hallmark is visceral involvement as well as skeletal lesions. The pulmonary changes are not specific by themselves but may resemble pulmonary fibrosis or focal infiltrates. (It may be helpful to study very carefully the corners of the chest radiograph in such a patient for clues such as hepatosplenomegaly or bone destruction and to examine the axilla and cervical regions for enlarged lymph nodes.)

Another manifestation of histiocytosis X not illustrated here is vertebra plana. If you see a patient with a wafer-thin vertebra, think of histiocytosis X.

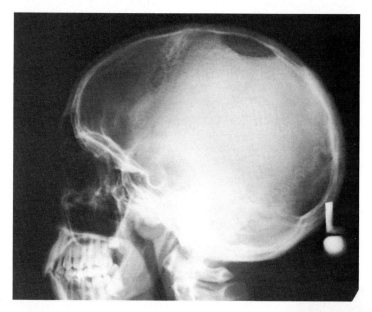

Figure 233. Peter H.

Peter Holloway is a 14 year old boy who had skull radiographs that were obtained for the evaluation of minimal head trauma. He was a healthy child with no previous surgery.

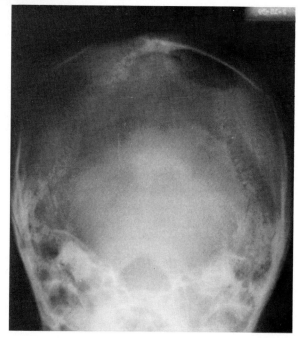

Figure 234. Peter H.

ANSWER

Do you have a problem with the interpretation of the holes in the parietal region of the skull? Be careful! The differential diagnosis includes not only histiocytosis, syphilis, and bilateral epidermoidomas but also a congenital defect known as parietal foramina. Parietal foramina are defects in the cranium caused by incomplete ossification of membranous bone. Small lesions are not at all uncommon, but large parietal foramina can be confused with other entities. The location, appearance, and clinical course establish the diagnosis—in our case—of parietal foramina.

EITHER YOU RECOGNIZE THIS CONDITION AT A GLANCE OR YOU HAVE NO IDEA WHAT IT IS

This case is an example of "pattern recognition," and once you've seen an example of it, you won't forget it.

Leo de O., age 9, was seen because of an asymmetrical face, and these radiographs were obtained. What is the diagnosis?

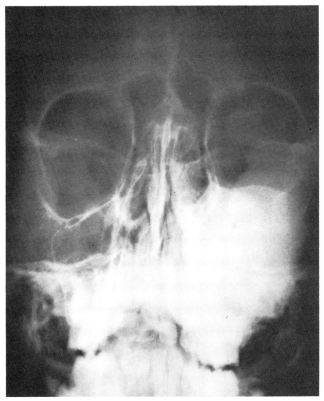

Figure 235. Leo de O.

ANSWER

The radiographs show a dense area of sclerosis involving the left sphenoid wing and maxillary bone. Bony encroachment has deformed the left maxillary sinus. No skin lesions were seen, and no other abnormalities of bone were identified on a skeletal survey.

This is **monostotic fibrous dysplasia.** In adults, it may be confused with the sclerotic phase of Paget's disease, blastic metastatic deposits, or, rarely, a very extensive meningioma. In childhood, craniofacial monostotic fibrous dysplasia is distinctive. It usually ceases activity at puberty, does not become malignant, and does not become transformed into polyostotic fibrous dysplasia or Albright's syndrome. In Albright's syndrome the bone changes of fibrous dysplasia are accompanied by café au lait spots and precocious puberty in females. This condition is distinct from *Leo de O.'s* monostotic fibrous dysplasia (but may perhaps be related metabolically).

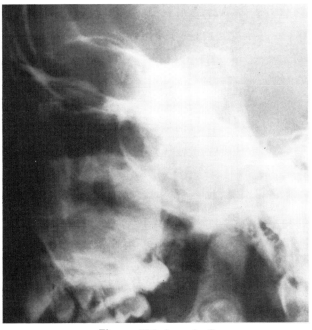

Figure 236. Leo de O.

VOMITING AND HEADACHE

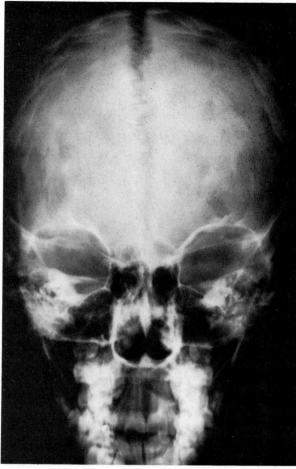

Figure 237. Stephen D.

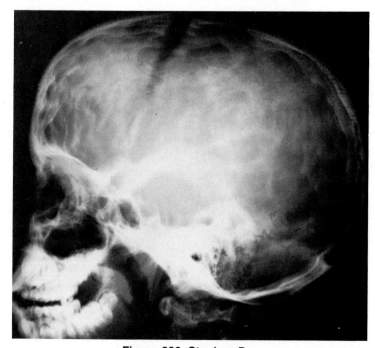

Figure 238. Stephen D.

Here is a 10 year old boy, **Stephen D.**, with truly disabling headaches accompanied by vomiting.

The pediatrician found bilateral papilledema and obtained skull radiographs (Figs. 237 and 238). These views are alarming because the sutures are obviously wide (diastatic). The lucent regions in the calvaria are not as useful a sign of increased intracranial pressure as the wide sutures because only slightly less marked lucencies are occasionally seen in the normal child. Note also that the dorsum is thinned and demineralized. This is a reliable sign of increased intracranial pressure, but in children below the age of 8 to 12 the still-open sutures are a more sensitive index of changes in intracranial pressure and will become abnormal before the sella does.

The problem, then, resolves itself into organization of a differential diagnosis of increased intracranial pressure in a 10 year old. We use the acronym TINC to help remember some of the causes of increased intracranial pressure.

The T stands for *trauma*. A child may have suffered trauma sufficiently severe to cause bilateral subdural hematomas without producing a skull fracture.

I is for *infection*, notably brain abscess, seen commonly in children with cyanotic congenital heart disease and in children with meningitis of any cause.

N is the first letter of *neoplasm*. Under this heading are included cerebellar medulloblastoma, brain stem and higher level gliomas, craniopharyngiomas, and papilloma of the choroid plexus.

The C of *congenital* is the last heading. Included in this group are aqueductal stenosis, Arnold-Chiari malformation (think of this if there is a meningomyelocele), and Dandy-Walker syndrome.

Actually, this scheme is not complete. For example, in what category would you place thrombosis of the sagittal sinus, or pseudotumor cerebri (benign increased intracranial pressure)?

ANSWER

Stephen D. had a complete work-up including a thorough history and physical examination as well as a lumbar puncture, complete blood count, blood culture, EEG, and a computed tomographic scan, which demonstrated aqueductal stenosis. The head size is within normal limits; however, the sutures are quite wide, indicating that the increased pressure is of recent onset. *Stephen* thus did not have typical congenital aqueductal stenosis with evidence of increased intracranial pressure starting at or before birth. Possibly, his increased pressure was acquired and secondary to hemorrhage or infection, although this is uncertain.

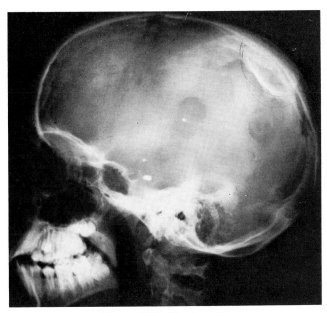

Figure 239. Stephen D.

A ventriculoperitoneal shunt was placed (Fig. 239). Notice that there is a radiopaque tubing with a dense marker at its tip. This is connected to a valve-flushing device combination that looks like a button in this illustration. The tubing is then tunneled through the superficial layers of the neck and chest into the peritoneal cavity, where the CSF is drained and reabsorbed.

The shunting procedure has resulted in diminished intracranial pressure, and the sutures and sella turcica appear normal. As the intracranial pressure decreases, sometimes a collection of blood develops in the epidural space. Normally, the intracranial pressure will tamponade such an accumulation, but the shunt device transmits the pressure to the peritoneal cavity and the epidural collection can expand. The calcified biconvex density seen in the posterior parietal region (Fig. 239 and detail in Fig. 240) is a calcified epidural hematoma. (The densities projected over the sella turcica are those of Pantopaque.)

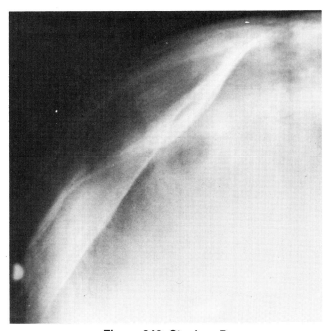

Figure 240. Stephen D.

MASS ON FOREHEAD

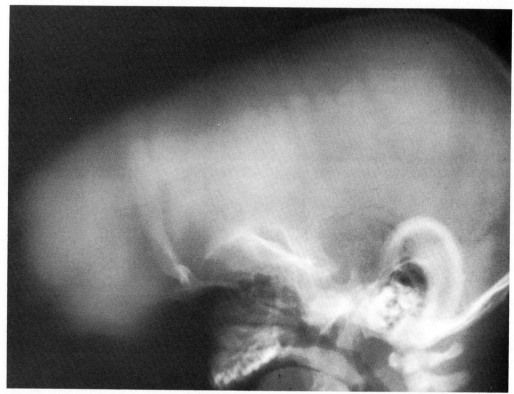

Figure 241. Baby Thomas

Baby Thomas was obviously malformed at birth, inasmuch as a huge soft tissue mass protruded anteriorly from the midline of the forehead. This mass was so large that the eyes were separated (hypertelorism), creating a most unusual appearance. This mass was found not to transilluminate with light. On the opposite page are two special procedures done prior to surgery.

What is your preoperative diagnosis?

ANSWER

The preoperative diagnosis was anterior encephalocele. One of the considerations helpful to the surgeons is the determination of the contents of the mass. Is there simply a small amount of dysplastic brain surrounded by fluid, or is the amount of brain much more substantial?

The ventriculogram (Fig. 242) demonstrates extension of a lateral ventricle into the mass. The amount of cerebral tissue seems substantial. The angiogram (Fig. 243) demonstrates the blood supply and also helps determine the amount of brain substance included in the encephalocele.

Surgery was performed utilizing an intracranial approach in the excision of the herniated and malformed brain. A tantalum plate covered the osseous defect. Later a diversionary procedure was necessary because of hydrocephalus (Fig. 244). *Baby Thomas* has done well since surgery, and he seems to have only moderate mental retardation.

Meningomyelocele is much more common than encephalocele. Among encephaloceles, furthermore, the anterior encephaloceles are much less common than the occipital encephaloceles. If an occipital encephalocele is present, not only cerebellum but also cerebral tissue may be herniated into the sac. A frontal encephalocele may protrude into the nose, simulating a nasal polyp, or may extend through the orbit, causing unilateral exophthalmos.

Surgery is indicated not only to prevent infection but also for removal of the unsightly mass.

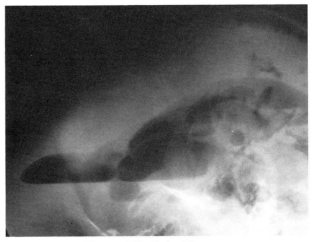

Figure 242. Baby Thomas

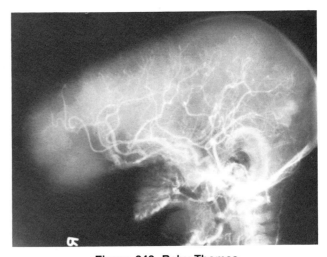

Figure 243. Baby Thomas

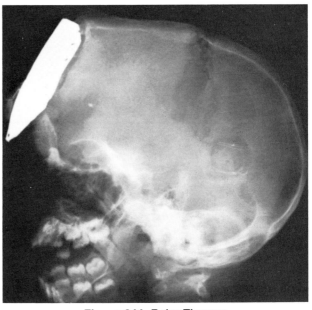

Figure 244. Baby Thomas

TWO INFANTS WITH HEAD TRAUMA

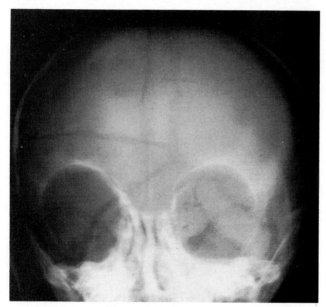

Figure 245. Tyrone F.

Tyrone F., age 4 months, was brought to the Emergency Room by his nearly hysterical mother. The history was obtained between self-recriminations and sobs; it seems that while *Tyrone* was having his diaper changed, he fell from the table onto the floor, striking his head.

Physical examination at the time of initial evaluation in the Emergency Room demonstrated that the child appeared well except for moderate soft tissue swelling in the right posterior parietal region. The pupils were of equal size, and both reacted to light. The remainder of the neurologic examination and the state of consciousness were normal. A set of skull radiographs was obtained and included Figures 245 and 246.

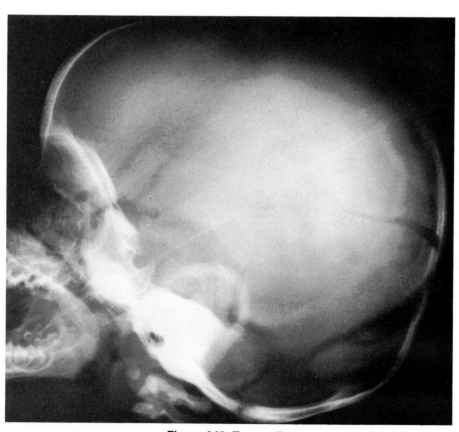

Figure 246. Tyrone F.

Patsy D., age 8 months, was also brought to the Emergency Room by her mother, who seemed quite calm and almost apathetic. She said the baby had been somewhat lethargic and had lost her appetite for the past week. She thought that the infant "might have hit her head" against the side of her crib a few days ago.

Physical examination showed an irritable infant who preferred to be left alone. There were ecchymoses over the head, legs, and buttocks. The pupils were equal in size and reacted to light, but the fundi could not be adequately examined because the child was too irritable. (The pediatrician did not use mydriatics to dilate the pupils because he would then have lost the ability to use inequality of pupils as a reliable sign of intracranial trauma.)

The sutures felt somewhat diastatic, and the anterior fontanelle was bulging. No skull fracture (or depressed skull fracture in particular) could be palpated. The skull radiographs were obtained because the history and physical examination raised the suspicion of *significant intracranial trauma.*

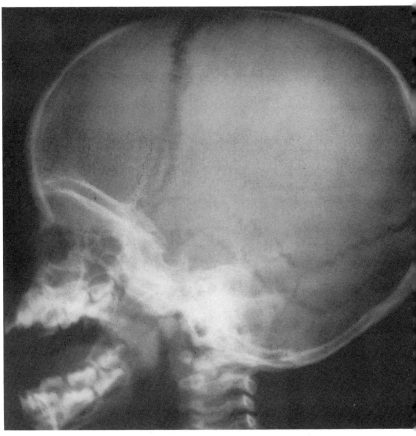

Figure 247. Patsy D.

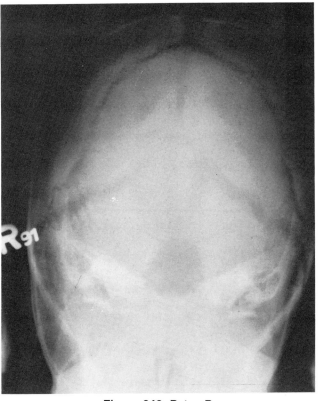

Figure 248. Patsy D.

ANSWERS

Tyrone F. has a skull fracture in the right posterior parietal region. No depression of the skull fracture fragments is seen, and the sutures appear normal.

Tyrone, in fact, appeared in no great distress. His state of consciousness was normal, as were his vital signs. He was not admitted to the hospital, and his parents were instructed to awaken him every two hours throughout the night to determine if he was asleep or if he had possibly lapsed into coma. They were also instructed how to evaluate pupil size and were told to bring the child back to the Emergency Room immediately if they detected any inequality in pupil diameter. However, *Tyrone* developed no signs of brain injury and has recovered completely.

Patsy D.'s radiographs (Figs. 247 and 248) show no skull fracture. Instead, there is a more ominous finding—diastasis of the sutures. Figure 248 is a Towne's view. The coronal suture, seen just superior to the foramen magnum on this radiograph, is greatly widened. The anterior fontanelle is superimposed on the middle of the occipital bone. The thin lucent lines radiating laterally from the foramen magnum are the synchondroses between the supraoccipital and exoccipital portions of the occipital bone. These are normal findings at this age.

Because of the presence of ecchymoses on other areas of the body, a skeletal survey was made to discover any evidence of trauma in the form of recent or healed fractures. No fractures were seen, but the history of hitting the head against the crib didn't seem compatible with a severe enough injury to produce diastatic sutures; therefore, the battered child syndrome (or "trauma X syndrome") was considered. In addition, the bulging fontanelle and the diastatic sutures were indications for computed tomography and bilateral subdural hematomas were found. Throughout the course of the next several days, the child had repeated subdural taps, where fluid was removed.

In retrospect, it seems likely that there had been definite head trauma during which the skull stopped moving immediately and the brain and dural attachments decelerated less rapidly. It is not surprising, then, that some of the vessels were torn, causing a collection of subdural blood, diastasis of the sutures, and bulging of the anterior fontanelle.

The day following *Patsy's* admission to the hospital, it was learned that a sibling had just been found dead at home after "falling down" a flight of stairs. The autopsy showed more than 60 ecchymoses on the child as well as liver and spleen lacerations. The evidence for battered child syndrome (see pages 180–181) was overwhelming, and *Patsy* was not sent home but was discharged to foster care.

The question of when radiographs of the skull are indicated in head trauma is clouded by the spurious concept of "medicolegal indications." It is argued by some physicians that if a skull series is not obtained and later something is found, a malpractice suit may result. This argument is even extrapolated to such a point that a skull series is obtained on all children with head trauma, whether mild, moderate, or severe. The result is that a tremendous number of children are radiographed with little expectation of yielding any important findings. The cost to parents and welfare agencies is astronomical, especially in proportion to the yield. A more economic approach, which reduces radiation exposure to the child, is the common sense approach: *If the sutures are palpably widened, if a depressed fracture is felt, if the child has evidence of severe head trauma or is unconscious, then radiographs are indicated, but for medical reasons, not legal reasons.* To allow legal considerations to dictate medical practice is unhealthy for the patient in terms of needless radiation exposure and is unnecessarily costly for society.

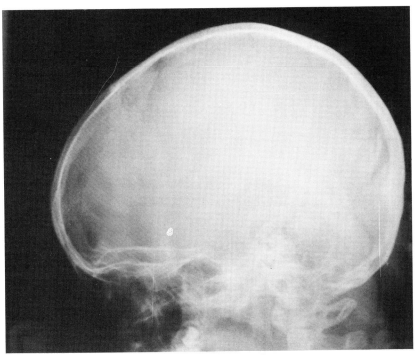

Figure 249. Seattle S.

Seattle S., a young but aspiring equestrian, was found unconscious in the paddock yard by her dressage coach. Can you help unravel the mystery of what happened by reading the images presented here?

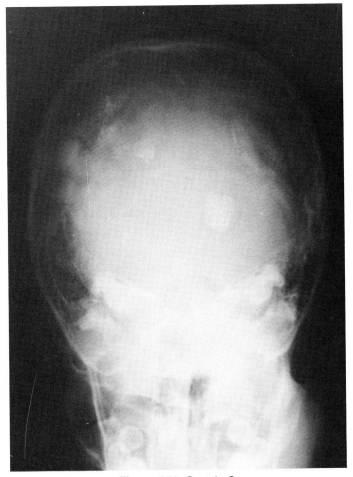

Figure 250. Seattle S.

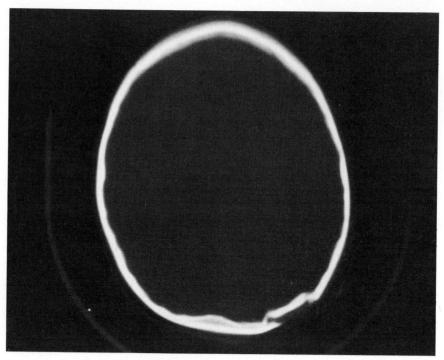

Figure 251. Seattle S.

ANSWER

First let's deal with those large, round densities overlying her skull—they represent pieces of gravel matted within *Seattle's* hair. Now, inspect the occipital bone on the left. Do you see the curved white line, which represents the overlapped cortical bone of a depressed skull fracture? This skull fracture is also seen clearly in the computed tomographic image obtained with a "bone window," in which imaging parameters are set so as to optimize bony detail. An important finding on *Seattle's* computed tomography scan was the absence of complicating intracranial bleeding at the fracture site.

So now you know that our young rider fell and was kicked in the head by her horse's hoof. Neurosurgical intervention will be required to elevate the depressed fragment, but we hope that *Seattle* will soon be back in the saddle again—next time wearing a suitable helmet!

Bone

TENDER SWELLING IN THE LEFT THIGH

Jill M., age 3 months, was brought to the Emergency Room by her mother, who stated, "My baby has a swollen leg." She could not think what might have caused this swelling, although she recalled that *Jill* seemed to have "twisted her leg in the crib" several days previously.

Physical examination showed a thin, almost emaciated baby obviously in pain. She held her left leg in flexion and resisted any attempt to move it. The swelling was confirmed, and radiographs of both extremities were obtained (Figs. 252 and 253).

ANSWER

The view of the left thigh shows a hard-to-see slender black line crossing the femur obliquely between the middle and lower thirds (compare with the child's normal right femur). This is a spiral fracture with no separation—a *recent* fracture because no callus is seen.

The comparison view of the right leg reveals a surprising finding. There is a fracture of the right tibia surrounded by abundant callus: hence, this is an *old* fracture. Notice also the irregularity of the most distal end of the tibia. This metaphyseal fraying is caused by avulsion of the insertion of the periosteum.

A skeletal survey was obtained and showed anterior compression of the fourth lumbar vertebra and, to a lesser degree, of the third lumbar vertebra (Fig. 254). The baby was admitted to the hospital with a diagnosis of *battered child syndrome*, i.e., child abuse.

As radiologists, we think of this di-

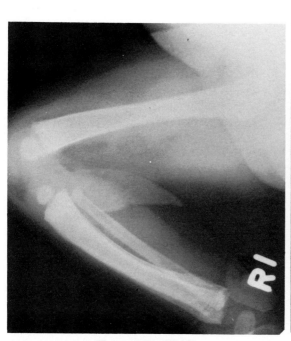

Figure 252. Jill M.

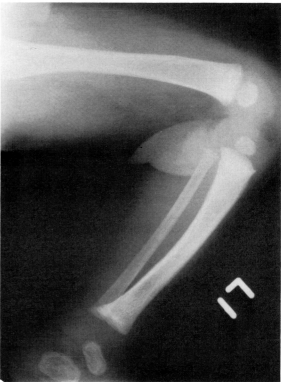

Figure 253. Jill M.

agnosis if we see the metaphyseal avulsions such as demonstrated in *Jill's* right tibia. If we have evidence for *fractures of different ages*, the battered child syndrome is almost certainly the explanation.

The question "Who did it?" is always a problem. This syndrome has been studied in great detail. Child batterers come from all levels of society. Only a small number are clearly psychotic. The vast majority of child abusers are not profoundly mentally ill, but one common thread that unites them is their exasperation and frustration with their children.

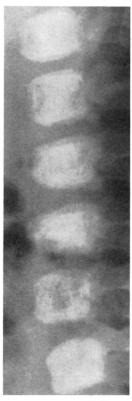

Figure 254. Jill M.

The battering commonly takes place when the baby is most frustrating: when he cries continuously and nothing will quiet him. At this point the baby is least satisfying, and he is rebuked for being "bad" by being physically abused.

The pediatrician recognizes the battered child by evidence of ecchymoses on the skin, contusions of the gums where a feeding bottle has been jammed into the mouth, hemorrhages into the retina secondary to cranial trauma, and so forth. A more subtle problem is to recognize the battered child with a less obvious manner of presentation, such as "failure to thrive" without apparent cause. Frequently, these children will thrive and gain weight when hospitalized, whereas the normal child usually does just the reverse.

Treatment should therefore begin with hospitalization. The parents are not confronted with the term "child batterer"; this would be counterproductive. Instead, therapy consists of trying to help the parents cope with their frustrations. Sometimes it is not safe to allow the child to return home, and a foster home must be sought, via the courts if necessary. At other times, gradual return of the child to the home environment can be achieved.

Jill's case was somewhat unusual, because the mother was mentally ill and *Jill* was initially sent to a chronic care facility while her mother received treatment. Only recently has the child returned home for three days a week. The remainder of the time she lives with a close relative. *Jill* is followed quite closely by a group caring for children with the battered child syndrome, and there has been no evidence of recurrence of abuse.

MORE PEDIATRIC TRAUMA . . .

Paula B., age 7, fell onto her right hand while skipping rope. AP and lateral radiographs of the wrist were obtained (Figs. 255 and 256).

ANSWER

Paula has a fracture of the distal end of the radius and ulna and anterior tilting of the distal fracture fragments. This suggests that her hand was held in volar flexion and was bent forward when she fell.

The fracture lines are not well seen because the fractures are impacted. However, the cortical buckling and deformity of alignment indicate that fractures of the radius and ulna have occurred.

This type of fracture is common and may be quite subtle. It is important to scrutinize the cortex of the distal radius and ulna for a minimal buckle before telling the parents that their child does not have a fracture.

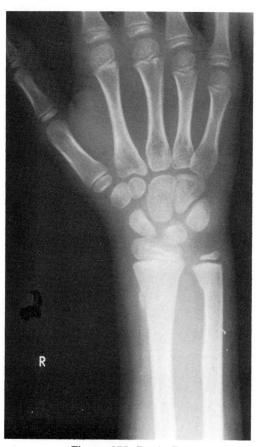

Figure 255. Paula B.

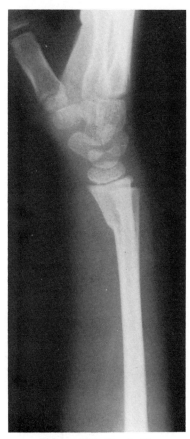

Figure 256. Paula B.

AND MORE . . .

Henry S., age 8 months, has been crawling all over his playpen with great vigor and has begun to use his legs more and more in an attempt to stand. Today, however, he stopped moving his left leg entirely, and an area of tenderness and erythema was noted. Radiographs of the region were obtained (Figs. 257 and 258).

ANSWER

Henry has a *"toddler's fracture,"* a spiral or oblique fracture of the distal left tibia. This type of injury may occur as the child is learning to walk. It frequently presents as a sudden and adamant refusal to walk or bear weight in an otherwise healthy child; the injury itself may have been unobserved. Sometimes the fractures are so occult that they cannot be seen on the initial radiographs but are visible on films made one to two weeks after the injury, when slight resorption of bone has occurred at the fracture margins and the periosteum has begun to lay down new bone. In *Henry's* case, it was not associated with any evidence of the battered child syndrome.

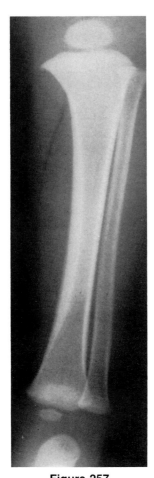

Figure 257.

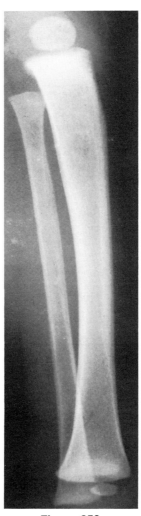

Figure 258.

Henry S.

A CONDITION THAT RADIOLOGICALLY RESEMBLES THE BATTERED CHILD SYNDROME

Pauline F., a 2 month old white female, was admitted to the hospital from the Outpatient Clinic because of swelling of the left wrist. She had been a 1700 gram premature baby, the product of a pregnancy that was complicated by a red, splotchy, cutaneous eruption in the mother during the third trimester. This was not investigated or treated.

The delivery was normal, and the baby remained in the hospital for three weeks gaining weight. She had done well at home until now.

Examination in the Outpatient Clinic showed *Pauline* to be a very small baby who held her left arm limp and cried continuously. Her liver and spleen were large. A lumbar puncture, CBC, urinalysis, and skeletal survey (Figs. 259, 260, and 261) were performed. A bone marrow aspirate clinched the diagnosis, although the radiographs were virtually specific for this condition, which is . . . ?

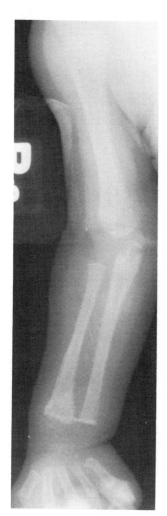

Figure 259.

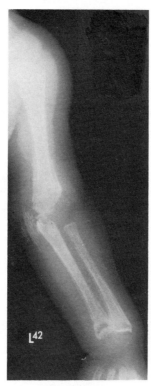

Figure 260.

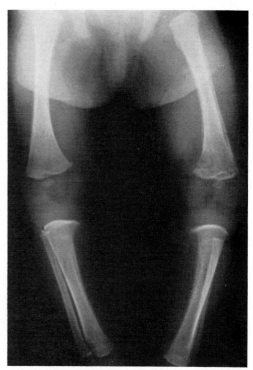

Figure 261.

ANSWER

The outstanding features of the radiographs are the spectacular periosteal reaction in multiple bones, the metaphyseal destruction, and the pathologic fractures. This is not the fine bilaterally symmetrical periosteal elevation that is sometimes seen in the normal newborn and young infant. Instead, this is a gross asymmetrical periosteal cloaking accompanied by metaphyseal destruction never seen in the benign periosteal reaction in the newborn.

As you suspected, *Pauline* has *congenital syphilis*. Sometimes in this condition, along the medial aspect of the proximal ends of the tibias, there may be symmetrical areas of destruction that are known as Wimberger's sign of congenital syphilis. The bone changes of congenital syphilis may also be seen in the calvarium and in the small bones of the hands and feet.

Because the diagnosis of congenital syphilis was extremely likely radiologically, the serologic test for syphilis was performed on the parents and the baby. Both the mother and *Pauline* had markedly positive titers—but these were not immediately available.

The bone marrow aspiration mentioned earlier revealed spirochetes characteristic of treponemes. This procedure is not one of the usual diagnostic tests in the evaluation of a patient with congenital syphilis; it was done here to exclude congenital leukemia or other neoplastic disease, which sometimes also causes widespread metaphyseal destruction.

In retrospect, it is clear that *Pauline's* limp arm was the pseudoparalysis of Parrot and was caused by severe pain resulting from metaphyseal destruction in the humerus. The hepatosplenomegaly is a consistent feature of congenital syphilis. Other findings seen in this condition that *Pauline* did not have include "snuffles," or rhinitis, skin eruption, and condylomata. However, she was anemic, a common feature of patients with congenital syphilis.

Pauline's mother's rash during the third trimester probably represented the cutaneous manifestations of secondary syphilis. Her disease was not diagnosed during the pregnancy, but after it became clear that her serologic test for syphilis was positive, she and the father were referred to the Public Health authorities for penicillin treatment and contact search. *Pauline* was treated with penicillin, also, and developed a febrile reaction and tachycardia characteristic of the Herxheimer reaction. This lasted for a short time and did not recur as treatment continued.

The child has been followed in the Outpatient Department. As of the last visit, *Pauline* had begun to move her left arm spontaneously, and the flagrant bone changes were reverting to normal.

THE CLASSICS

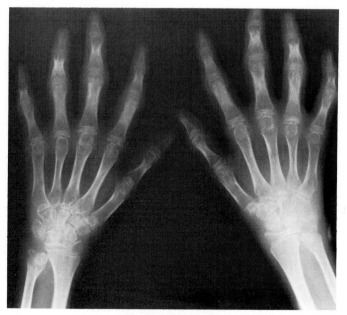

Figure 262. Tina L.

Here are **the classics,** bone radiographs that time has served to sanctify and examiners to dignify by inclusion in all sorts of quiz presentations, examinations, and Boards. Topics that have been previously covered in *Exercises in Diagnostic Radiology, Volume 3, Bone,* will not be covered in as much detail here.

Tina L., a 7 year old retired concert pianist, was unable to sign her unemployment compensation check because of stiff fingers. This radiograph was obtained (Fig. 262).

Phillip D., a 1 year old food faddist, had a skeletal survey to confirm the clinical impression—which was . . . ? (This is an ancient case; today, we would shield the gonads.)

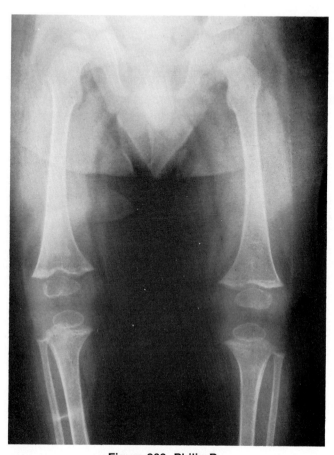

Figure 263. Philip D.

Mac W., age 1, is another food faddist (Fig. 264).

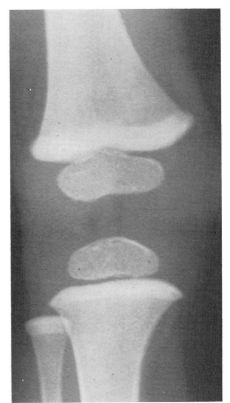

Tom S., age 9, might have been fed a very special diet that would have caused the bones to develop this radiographic appearance. However, he was fed a normal diet but developed these bone changes anyway (Figs. 265 and 266).

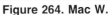
Figure 264. Mac W.

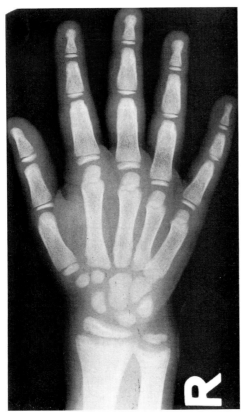
Figure 265. Tom S.

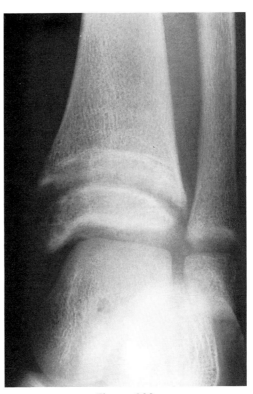
Figure 266.

ANSWERS

Tina L.'s hand radiographs demonstrate soft tissue swelling surrounding the proximal interphalangeal joints. In addition, the bones show generalized osteoporosis (reduced bone density). The margins of the carpal bones are irregular, indistinct, and reflect extensive bone destruction.

Tina has *juvenile rheumatoid arthritis (JRA)*. Her symptoms began with stiffness in both hands. (A somewhat more classic presentation would have been fever, pain, and stiffness in the larger joints such as the knees or elbows.) Earlier radiographs showed only soft tissue swelling, but the current films show advanced changes of juvenile rheumatoid arthritis.

The radiographic changes are caused by chronic inflammation, with thickening of the synovium that surrounds the joints and destruction of the cartilage and eventually the bone. Hyperemia accompanies the inflammatory changes and is responsible for the deossification. Advanced bone age may occur in JRA; it is the hyperemia that is thought to cause this.

Tina has been treated with moderate success with aspirin and steroids and physical therapy. The deformity and limitation of range of motion of the fingers and hands seem to be at least stable at the present time.

Philip D. has extremely osteoporotic bones. The appearance of these bones has been stated to resemble ground glass. The epiphyses have a cortical margin that is well defined and relatively radiodense. This is a distinctive feature of this condition. The metaphyses are flared. Fractures occurring through the zones of provisional calcification result in chipped-off "corners."

Philip has *scurvy*. This is caused by vitamin C (ascorbic acid) deficiency and is manifest clinically by bleeding gums and tenderness in the legs. *Philip* had been fed exclusively boiled cow's milk without vitamin supplementation. Cow's milk has considerably less vitamin C than breast milk, and boiling it reduces the vitamin C content even further. When treatment was begun with vitamin supplementation, calcification of the periosteal hematomas occurred (Fig. 267).

Mac W.'s bone radiographs demonstrate the dense metaphyseal bands associated with lead ingestion. (One caution, however: The normal patient may have dense femoral and tibial metaphyses, especially around age 2 years. The proximal fibular metaphysis never is this dense normally, however.) Other reliable places to scan in evaluating a patient for lead ingestion include the distal ulna, the inferior border of the scapula, and the iliac crest—in other words, sites of rapid endochondral ossification.

The dense metaphyseal band does not represent locally deposited lead; it is secondary to the effect of lead, which alters the trabecular architecture of the newly formed bone. It has been stated that the lead interferes with the balance between deposition and resorption of bone. There is continued deposition of bone, which appears radiologically as a dense metaphyseal band.

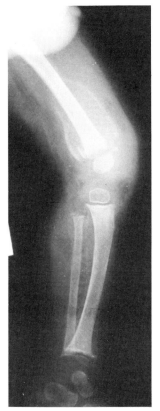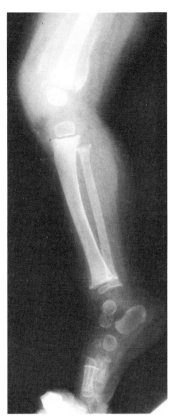

Figure 267. Philip D.

Mac W. had recently eaten lead-containing paint, which appeared as radiopaque debris in the colon (Fig. 268). The colon was emptied of its poisonous contents, and courses of chelation progressively removed lead from the body.

The bone disease is almost incidental and causes the patient virtually no problems. It's the CNS that takes the blow and the bones that give the clue.

Tom S.'s radiographs show widening of the growth plates of the radius and ulna, accompanied by cupping and fraying of the normally smooth borders of the metaphyses. Defective calcification of the osteoid is reflected radiologically by increased distance between the metaphysis and epiphysis.

Tom has vitamin D–resistant rickets, an inherited unresponsiveness to normal quantities of vitamin D. His diet contained a normal amount of vitamin D. When *Tom* received a diet massively supplemented with vitamin D, healing occurred.

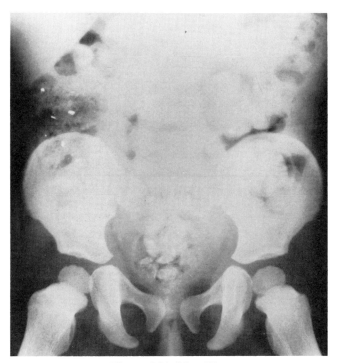

Figure 268. Mac W.

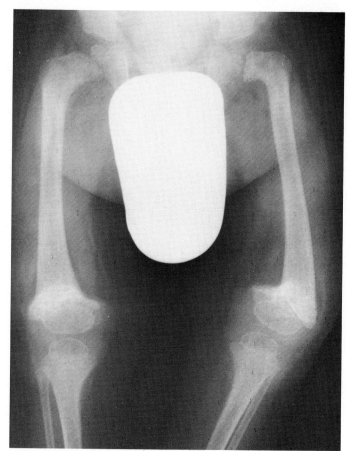

Figure 269. Tom S.

Tom S.'s chest radiograph (Fig. 270) shows marked expansion of the anterior ribs, the radiologic counterpart of the physical finding known as rachitic rosary, which is due to accumulation of nonossified osteoid at the costochondral junction.

The pelvic and lower extremity radiograph shows many features of rickets. The rachitic bone has resulted in a decrease in the angle between the femoral neck and femoral shaft, known as coxa vara. The bony trabeculae are coarsened, the cartilage plates are widened, and the distal femoral metaphyses are cupped. All of the bones are demineralized.

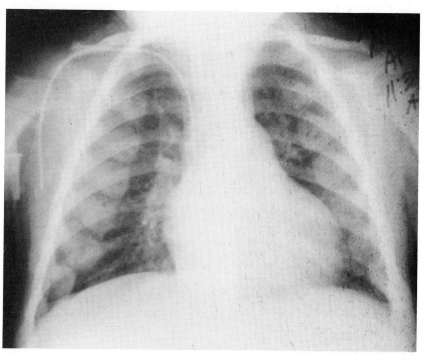

Figure 270. Tom S.

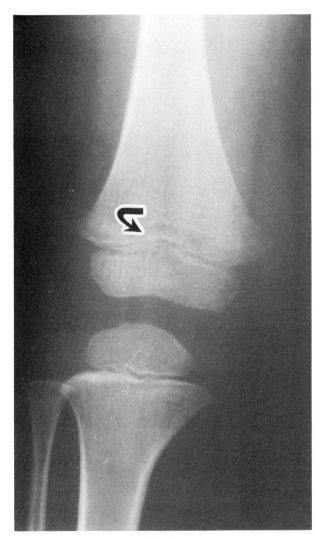

George Whitehall is a 3 year old boy with arthralgias that were somewhat suggestive of JRA. This anteroposterior knee radiograph was obtained as part of *George's* work-up.

Figure 271. George W.

ANSWER

If no finding leaps out at you, look closely at the metaphyseal portions of the distal femur and proximal tibia. There is a black or radiolucent line just beneath a white line (arrow). These lines of increased and decreased radiodensity are the most common bone findings in the disease *George* has—leukemia. The best place to look for these findings is in areas of rapid bone growth, that is, the femur and tibia at the knee and the distal radius and ulna at the wrist.

These bone changes are probably not caused by leukemic infiltration but rather represent abnormal ossification of bone. (This finding, by the way, is also seen in severe malnutrition.)

Other bone findings seen in leukemia are diffuse lytic lesions, periosteal new bone formation, and, rarely, osteoblastic lesions.

Clinically, leukemia may masquerade as JRA or as metastatic neuroblastoma. The radiographic finding of transverse bands of increased and decreased radiodensity should quickly suggest leukemia, and an evaluation conducted with that diagnosis in mind is the prime consideration.

THE CLASSICS, PART TWO

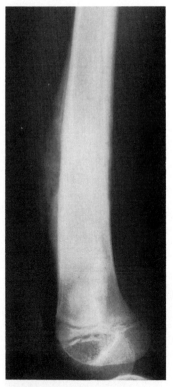

Figure 272. Christopher T.

Christopher T., age 8, had suffered a trivial injury while playing baseball. He had thought that he had a "charley horse," but because the pain didn't diminish and *Christopher* began to limp, his mother brought him to the pediatrician. Included here is one of the radiographs of the thigh area (Fig. 272).

Cheryl S., 14 years old, appeared quite ill. For approximately two weeks she had pain and soft tissue swelling in the region of the midportion of the right humerus. Recently the swelling and tenderness became more than she could bear, and she was seen by her pediatrician, who admitted her immediately to the hospital with the provisional diagnosis of osteomyelitis (Fig. 273).

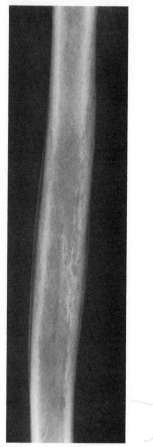

Figure 273. Cheryl S.

Seth P. was 17 years old when these radiographs were obtained (Figs. 274 and 275). His diagnosis had been established three years earlier on the basis of a cervical lymph node biopsy. He had received treatment, but back pain and symptoms of nausea, vomiting, and decreasing appetite had recently occurred. These radiographs were followed by an upper gastrointestinal and small bowel series (Fig. 277). What are the possible diagnoses? Has *Seth* had back surgery?

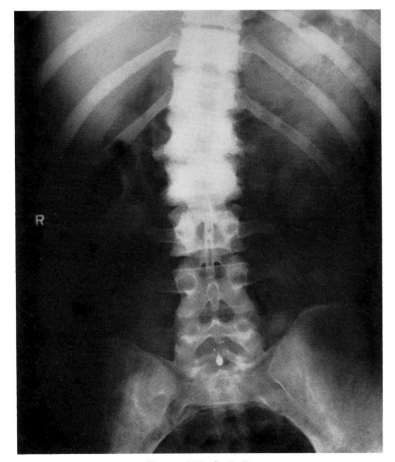

Figure 274. Seth P.

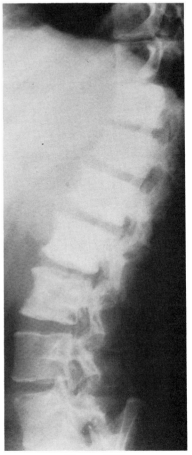

Figure 275.

ANSWERS

The radiograph of *Christopher's* femur (Fig. 272) shows an increased bone density of the distal half of the femur. Anteriorly, there is elevation and disruption of the periosteum accompanied by layers of periosteal reaction. Notice that there is tumor formation in the soft tissue. These are the findings of osteogenic sarcoma. Whether the increased density in the lower femur is caused by tumor new bone formation or by bone reaction to the neoplastic process is not known.

This malignant bone tumor has a poor prognosis regardless of treatment. *Christopher* had an amputation of his leg; however, he developed lung metastases several months after surgery and died less than one year after the osteogenic sarcoma was discovered.

Cheryl S.'s clinical condition suggested osteomyelitis. She had the classic findings of inflammation: swelling, heat, redness, and loss of function. The radiograph of the humerus (Fig. 273) shows a mottled appearance to the mid-diaphyseal region, indicating that a destructive process has permeated the bone. This area of involvement is accompanied by lamellae of periosteal reaction anteriorly and posteriorly. The lamellae of periosteum are sometimes referred to as having an "onion peel" appearance.

Because of the clinical impression of osteomyelitis, *Cheryl* was operated upon and the lesion was drained and biopsied. The pathology report was *Ewing's sarcoma*!

Ewing's sarcoma is a malignant bone tumor thought to arise from blood-forming elements. Its syptoms, signs, and radiographic appearance resemble osteomyelitis to a striking degree. The treatment of choice is radiotherapy. The prognosis is better than with osteogenic sarcoma, and *Cheryl* has just completed her radiotherapy. There is not yet any evidence of metastases in the lungs or elsewhere, but it is still too soon to predict whether the radiotherapy was successful.

The differential diagnosis of periosteal reaction is important. Below (Fig. 276) is a child with periosteal reaction seen along the lateral aspect of the lower femora. This child has leukemia. Here is a list of *some conditions that may cause periosteal reaction:*

Benign

1. Osteomyelitis
2. Bone infarct (think of sickle cell anemia)
3. Caffey's disease (infantile cortical hyperostosis)
4. Treated scurvy (caused by ossification of subperiosteal bleeding)
5. Hypertrophic pulmonary osteoarthropathy (think of cystic fibrosis)
6. Osteoid osteoma
7. Gaucher's disease (not common)
8. Trauma
9. Eosinophilic granuloma (histiocytosis X)

Malignant

1. Osteogenic sarcoma
2. Ewing's sarcoma
3. Leukemia
4. Other primary and metastatic tumors of bone

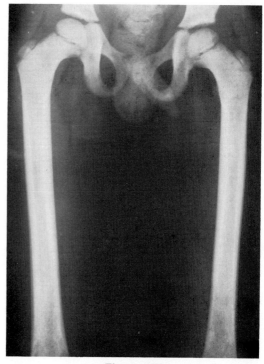

Figure 276.

Seth's spine radiographs (Figs. 274 and 275) show that the eleventh and twelfth thoracic vertebrae as well as the first and second lumbar vertebrae are exceedingly radiodense. The third lumbar vertebra has patchy areas of increased radiodensity within it. The lucent area seen on the AP projection extending from the center of T 11 to L 2 is caused by surgery—a laminectomy. *Seth* has Hodgkin's disease, which has involved the spine and caused spinal cord compression. A laminectomy was needed to decompress the spinal cord.

Blastic changes in the bone are uncommon in the pediatric population. However, they are seen in Hodgkin's disease, medulloblastoma, osteogenic sarcoma, and occasionally in leukemia. Lytic metastatic deposits, on the other hand, are seen very frequently, especially in neuroblastoma and leukemia.

Seth's small bowel series (Fig. 277) demonstrated separation of loops of small bowel accompanied by fixation and imprint formation or indentation on the serosal surface. This is caused by involvement of the mesentery with Hodgkin's disease. The initial chest radiograph (Fig. 278) revealed massive mediastinal lymph node enlargement. The diagnosis of Hodgkin's disease was proved by cervical lymph node biopsy. *Seth* had radiotherapy and chemotherapy.

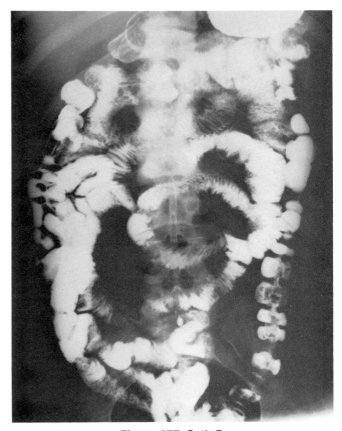

Figure 277. Seth P.

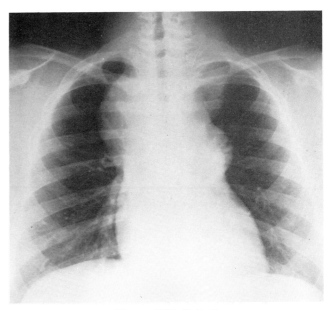

Figure 278. Seth P.

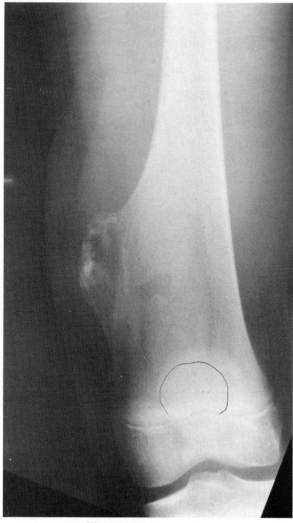

Figure 279. Teresa B.

Teresa B., an 11 year old girl, became alarmed when she felt a lump in her thigh. Her pediatrician requested the radiograph presented here. What is the name of this lesion, and what would you tell *Teresa* and her parents?

ANSWER

Teresa's radiograph shows an osseous lesion projecting from the medial surface of the distal femur. The cortex of the mass is continuous with the cortex of the femur, and its "cap" has discontinuous areas of nonhomogeneous radiopacity.

Teresa need not be alarmed, as she has a benign bone tumor that is known as an exostosis or osteochondroma. These tumors are most commonly detected in the long tubular bones of adolescent children. An interesting feature of osteochondromata is that they tend to point away from adjacent joints.

Sarcomatous degeneration is a very uncommon complication of solitary osteochondromata and occurs in less than one per cent of patients. However, if the patient complains of local pain or if the lesion grows after closure of the growth plates, malignancy should be suggested.

Osteochondromata may also occur as multiple lesions. This condition is inherited as an autosomal dominant trait and has an incidence of malignant degeneration of about five per cent.

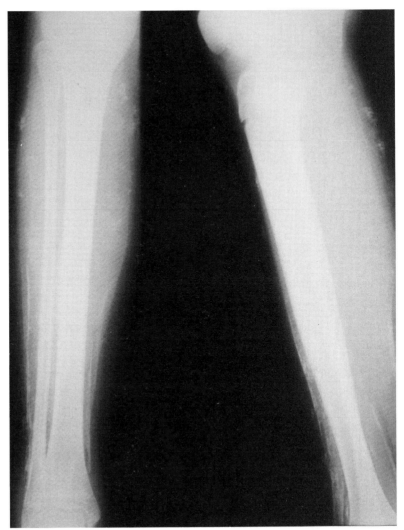

This radiograph of the lower extremities of a 10 year old girl, **Bonnie White,** shows soft tissue calcifications that are characteristic of a generalized disease process. What is the diagnosis?

Figure 280. Bonnie W.

ANSWER

Bonnie has subcutaneous calcifications that appear as linear plaques and that tend to follow the facial planes. Our patient has dermatomyositis, and these soft tissue changes are classic! In other cases one may see muscular atrophy and reduced mineralization of the bone because of weakness and restricted ambulation.

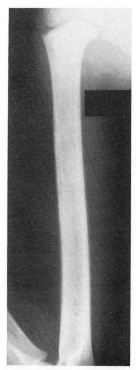

Figure 281. Shawanda T., June 21

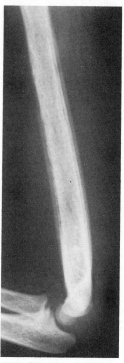

Figure 282. Shawanda T., June 30

More Periosteal Reaction . . .

Shawanda T., age 7, a black girl with sickle cell anemia, was seen because of pain in the right arm of two days' duration.

Radiographs of her arm were taken on June 21 (Fig. 281) and showed soft tissue swelling, expansion of the marrow space (thinned cortex), and fine periosteal reaction. These radiologic features are consistent with a bone infarct, and *Shawanda* was admitted to the hospital. A bone marrow aspiration documented *Salmonella* osteomyelitis. On June 30, a second radiograph was obtained, which showed permeative, moth-eaten changes in the humerus accompanied by a more extensive periosteal reaction. With antibiotic therapy, the child slowly improved.

Here is a common problem: the differentiation of bone infarct from osteomyelitis in sickle cell anemia. Radiologically these conditions may appear exactly the same, and clinical and bacteriologic factors must form the basis for their differentiation. Children with sickle cell anemia are subject to both illnesses. The osteomyelitis is often caused by one of the *salmonellae*.

Other bone changes in sickle cell anemia include expansion of the medullary space caused by an increased volume of red marrow. There is an exaggerated prominence to the bony trabeculae. The vertebrae have a characteristic appearance on the lateral view that resembles the child's toy known as Lincoln Logs. There is also an increased incidence of aseptic necrosis of the femoral head and other epiphyses. A curious entity is the "hand-foot" syndrome, in which there are infarcts of the small bones of the hands and feet. Radiographs show periosteal reaction of the small tubular bones.

And Still More . . .

Jack C., age 3 months, had been irritable for about four days. He had also had a low-grade fever and soft-tissue swelling that surrounded the mandible and both forearms.

The AP view of the mandible shows a "new" layer of bone. Normally the roots of the molars are within 2 or 3 millimeters of the exterior of the mandible in this age group. Here the new bone has almost doubled the thickness of the mandible (Fig. 283).

There is another finding seen on this radiograph: periosteal cloaking of the left clavicle. Similar findings are present in the radius and ulna on each side (Fig. 284).

These are the radiographic findings of **infantile cortical hyperostosis,** or **Caffey's disease.** This condition occurs in infants under age 5 months. The etiology is unknown, but infection, allergy, toxins, drugs, and hereditary factors have been suggested. The bones most commonly involved are the mandible, clavicle, ribs, and long bones of the extremities. Changes of infantile cortical hyperostosis are not seen in the phalanges or in the vertebral bodies.

Radiographically, the differential diagnosis includes the trauma X (battered child) syndrome and infection, such as syphilis. Usually the pattern of bone involvement (the mandible is most frequently involved) suggests the correct diagnosis.

Although most patients heal without specific therapy, steroids have been used. Some patients may develop a chronic form of this condition and demonstrate bony bridges between the ribs or radius and ulna.

The disease seems to be less common now than in the 1950s, for unknown reasons.

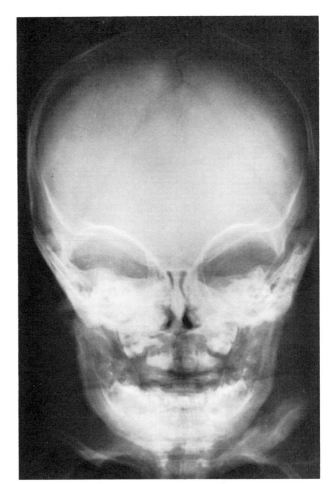

Figure 283. Jack C.

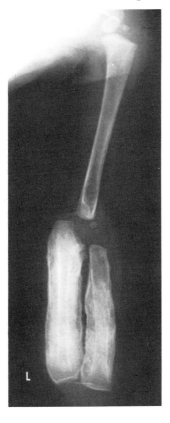
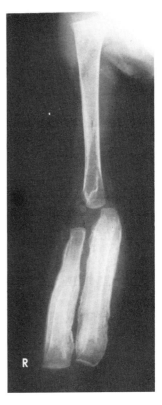

Figure 284. Jack C.

NOW HOW ABOUT THIS PATIENT?

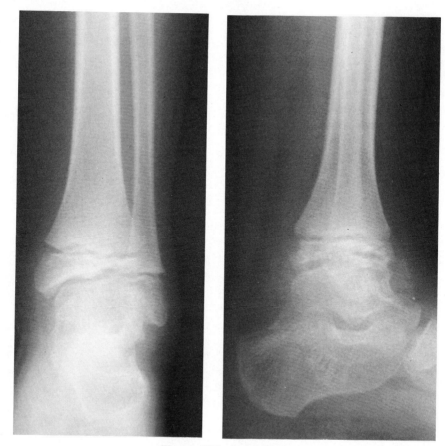

Figure 285. Judah R.

Judah R., a 4 year old boy, has bruising, swelling, and pain about the left ankle, which began after he started to walk. What are the roentgen observations, and what is your diagnosis?

ANSWER

There is soft tissue swelling about the ankle accompanied by an irregular appearance of the articular surfaces of the tibiotalar joint. With the stated history, these findings should suggest recurrent hemorrhage into the joint caused by a bleeding disorder. The hemorrhage causes synovial hypertrophy, and this in turn results in destruction of the joint.

Judah R. has Factor VIII deficiency (classic hemophilia) and hemophiliac arthritis.

LIMPING WITH PAIN IN THE RIGHT HIP

Dick C., age 3., was observed to be limping for about three days. Initially, his mother thought that he might have had pain in the right knee, but subsequently she thought that the pain was centered in the right hip. The pediatrician found slight tenderness in the hip region and limitation of range of motion accompanied by muscle spasm. He obtained these radiographs (Figs. 286 and 287).

The AP and "frog leg" lateral hip views show flattening of the right femoral epiphysis, with irregular areas of rarefaction between areas of increased bone density. The right femoral neck is slightly broader than the left.

This is Legg-Perthes disease, which is ischemic necrosis of the capital femoral epiphysis. This condition is more common in boys. Its peak incidence is about age 7, but children as young as 2 years old have been seen with Legg-Perthes disease. Ischemic necrosis of the hip is also seen in association with Gaucher's disease, sickle cell anemia, hypothyroidism, steroid therapy, and in late stages of treatment of congenital hip dislocation.

The early radiologic manifestations of Legg-Perthes disease are an increase in the apparent joint space and fullness of periarticular soft tissue planes. A subchondral lucency then develops in the epiphysis. This lucency is crescent-shaped and in the next stage is followed by areas of dense bone separated by lucent areas composed of fibrous tissue. The femoral head appears to be dissolving into several fragments. It is flattened, and the femoral neck is widened. When repair begins, gradual reconstruction of shape is seen, with diminution in size of the lucent areas.

Notice the left hip in the frog leg projection. There is a lucent crescent in the joint space between the acetabulum and the epiphysis. This is gas that accu-

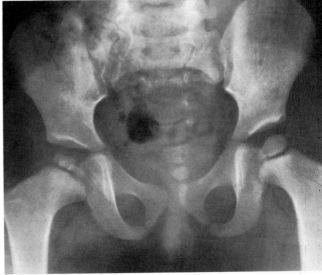

Figure 286. Dick C.

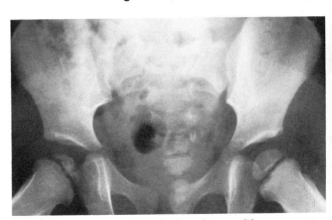

Figure 287. Dick C., frog leg position

mulated in the joint space as *Dick's* hip was gently manipulated into the frog leg position. Caused by diminished pressure in the joint during manipulation, this gas outlines the thickness of the articular cartilage. This is a "gas arthrogram" or the "vacuum phenomenon." The formation of a gas arthrogram in the hip has no specific significance by itself.

Adele Click is a 10 month old girl with asymmetrical gluteal creases. Her pediatrician thinks that she has a dislocation of the right hip. Do you agree?

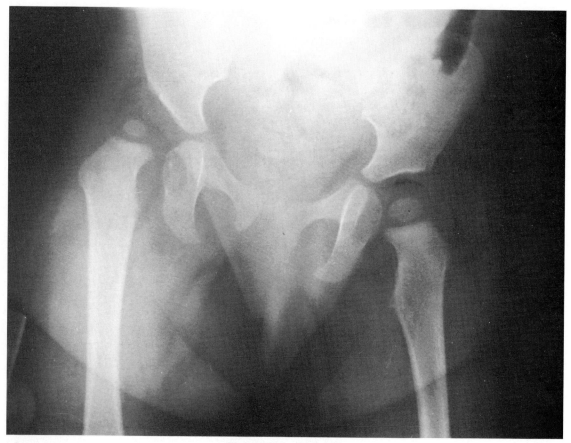

Figure 288. Adele C.

ANSWER

Note the asymmetry of the gluteal creases; the right crease is more superior than the left. Also observe that the right capital femoral epiphysis is smaller than the left, that the slope of the right acetabular roof is steeper than the left, and that the right hip is dislocated. These findings are a classic triad seen in congenital hip dislocation (CDH), a condition that is much more common in girls than in boys and that involves the left hip many times more frequently than the right.

The etiology of CDH is debated even at this time, but it is probably a result of ligamentous laxity. Prompt recognition and treatment in the neonatal period are important to reduce the morbidity related to this disorder. Since in the neonate with a dislocated or dislocatable hip the capital femoral epiphysis is not yet ossified, the acetabulum is not yet dysplastic, and the hip is often little displaced from its normal location, the diagnosis usually depends on clinical and not radiologic evaluation.

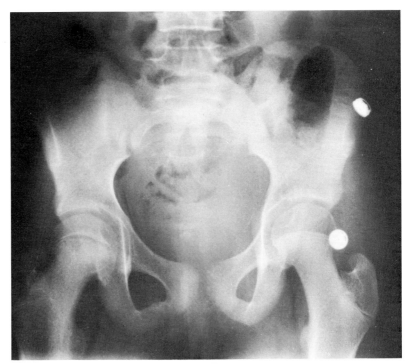

Figure 289. F. G. M.

This is **Fredericka G. Moses,** an overweight 13 year old girl who is being evaluated for pain in the right hip.

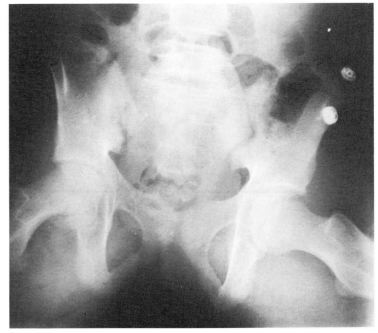

Figure 290. F. G. M.

ANSWER

Start by looking at the frog leg view of the hips (Fig. 290). May we also suggest that you use the normal left hip as a guide for appropriate anatomic relationships? Now notice that the anterior and posterior corners of the right capital femoral epiphysis do not align with the corners of the metaphysis of the femoral neck. The femoral head has "slipped," and *Fredericka* has a condition that goes by the very imaginative name of slipped capital femoral epiphysis (SCFE).

SCFE is more common in boys than in girls, more common in blacks than in whites, and more common in overweight than in normal weight children. It is important to note that about 25 per cent of patients have bilateral SCFE. However, if a child is seen initially with bilateral SCFE, look very carefully at the radiographs to exclude rickets. (And remember that a common cause of rickets in older children is renal failure.)

Fredericka should not walk from your x-ray department to the orthopedic surgery clinic because the degree of slip may increase. So put her in a wheelchair or on a bed and send her on her way, which will include a trip to the operating room, where surgical pinning will be performed to stabilize the femoral head to prevent further slippage.

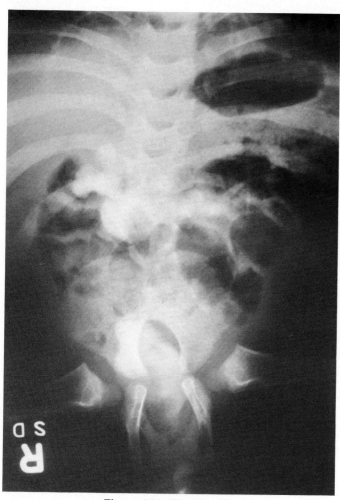

Figure 291. Timothy N.

Timothy Nobottom is a 4 year old boy who was born with a severe deformity of his lower body. What is the pertinent roentgen observation, and what is the ailment that this child's mother might have?

ANSWER

Timothy has agenesis of his lumbosacral spine. Do you see that his iliac bones articulate with each other? Youngsters with this anomaly, which is termed the caudal regression syndrome, usually have a neurogenic rectum and bladder with associated chronic urinary tract infections and orthopedic abnormalities. His mother has diabetes mellitus, which is present in 20 per cent of mothers of children with sacral agenesis.

Jack Back is a 15 year old boy who complains of pain between his shoulder blades. Can you make a diagnosis from the radiograph illustrated here?

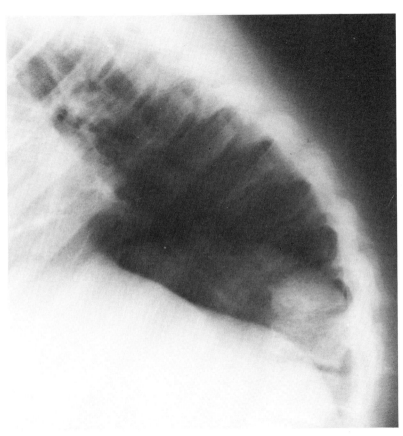

Figure 292. Jack B.

ANSWER

The radiographic observations are kyphosis, or abnormal backward curvature of the thoracic spine, anterior wedging of multiple vertebral bodies, and indentations on the end-plates of the vertebral bodies. All together, these findings constitute the changes seen in juvenile kyphosis, or Scheuermann's disease. The etiology of the disease is unknown. However, the indentations on the vertebral end-plates are caused by disc herniations called Schmorl's nodes and are thought to be related to trauma.

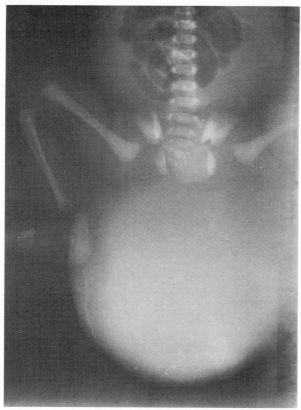

Figure 293. F. Buxton

Fletcher Buxton was born with a huge mass protruding from his buttocks. Can you propose a diagnosis?

ANSWER

The large soft-tissue mass demonstrated on the radiograph in Figure 293 contains faintly visible calcification and represents a sacrococcygeal teratoma. These lesions may contain a variety of tissues, including fat, teeth, bowel, or elements of the central nervous system. Most lesions are benign, but owing to significant malignant potential they are all removed in the newborn period.

By the way, did you notice the bowel obstruction caused by the intrapelvic position of the mass, which has displaced and compressed the gut?

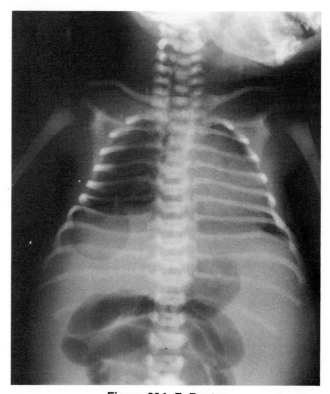

Figure 294. F. Buxton

Annette Pamplemousse is an 11 year old girl who has recently developed weakness in her legs accompanied by positive neurologic findings. Look at the frontal and lateral view of the spine. What is your diagnosis?

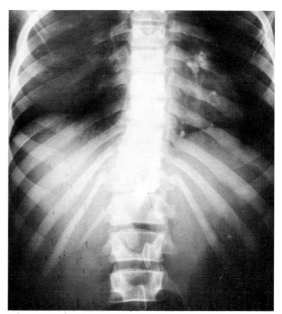

Figure 295. Annette P.

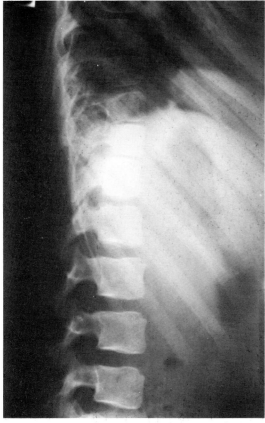

Figure 296. Annette P.

ANSWER

The roentgen findings include an abnormal bony spur at the T 11/T 12 level, neural arch defects, and abnormalities in shape and size of the vertebral bodies. The spur is most important because it divides and tethers the spinal cord into two parts at the midsagittal plane. As the child grows, tension, which may cause neurologic impairment, is placed on the spinal cord.

This condition is known as diaste-matomyelia, and if you know about it you have already learned 50 per cent of the required knowledge for this page of the book. (If you can *spell* diastematomyelia, you know 100 per cent . . . .)

The spur may consist of fibrous or cartilaginous tissue rather than bone. For further evaluation of a patient with diastematomyelia prior to surgery, a myelogram or metrizamide-enhanced computed tomography is performed.

SKELETAL DYSPLASIAS

For many pediatric radiologists, the most difficult conditions to categorize are the skeletal dysplasias. This group of maladies comprises the inborn diseases that are reflected in unusual patterns of bone size and/or shape. The radiologist soon learns that it is necessary but not sufficient to memorize one pattern of bone malformation for each disease. The patterns change as the patient grows. In addition, in some of the dysplasias there is a spectrum of involvement from mild to severe. In general, it is a sterile (and frequently boring) exercise to try to deduce from a set of radiographs alone the condition responsible for the changes. The history, physical examination, and genetic pattern in the family, studied together with the radiographs, make an exciting diagnostic challenge, and in this context a few of the more common skeletal dysplasias will be presented here.

What do we mean by skeletal dysplasias? In general, they are inherited, although many occur by spontaneous mutation. Rubin has suggested that the pattern of altered bone growth reflects the site of major derangement, such as the epiphysis, growth plate, metaphysis, or diaphysis.

In this section, we also discuss and illustrate some of the **mucopolysaccharidoses (MPS)**. There are at least seven conditions included in this general category: Hurler syndrome (MPS IH), Hunter syndrome (MPS II), Sanfilippo syndrome (MPS III), Morquio syndrome (MPS IV), Scheie syndrome (MPS IS), Maroteaux-Lamy syndrome (MPS VI), and Sly syndrome (MPS VII). These conditions have in common excessive storage in many tissues and urinary excretion of certain mucopolysaccharides.

There is another group of connective tissue disorders that show altered bone growth and/or mineralization, which, together with the clinical information, form a recognizable pattern. This group of diseases includes Marfan's syndrome, homocystinuria, and fibrodysplasia ossificans progressiva.

Why put so much effort into cataloguing such rare and apparently hopeless conditions? The answer depends upon one's orientation. For the researcher studying cartilage growth, the patients with achondroplasia, hypochondroplasia, and achondrogenesis are models of abnormal cartilage cell growth. For the clinician caring for the patient with homocystinuria, it is quite important to know that arteriograms are to be avoided: patients with homocystinuria develop thromboses and may die. For the genetic counselor, it is important to differentiate diastrophic dwarfism, which is inherited as a recessive trait, from achondroplasia, an autosomal dominant condition.

Last, for the patient, evidence is accumulating that metabolic abnormalities may be correctable in at least some of these conditions. For example, the altered metabolism of fibroblasts from patients with the Hurler syndrome is corrected by adding the missing enzyme to the culture fluid. The next problem is to find an effective way of administering the enzyme to the patient.

THE CLINICAL APPEARANCE OF FOUR DWARFS

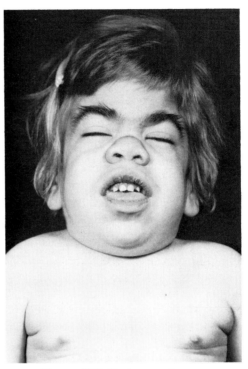

Figure 297. Hurler syndrome

The following illustrations are of dwarfs with skeletal dysplasias, including the Hurler syndrome, or MPS IH (Fig. 297); the Morquio syndrome, or MPS IV (Fig. 298); achondroplasia (Fig. 299); and pycnodysostosis (Fig. 300). (These are not the same patients whose skeletal surveys are seen on the following pages.)

The *Hurler syndrome* is inherited as an autosomal recessive trait. The patient illustrated here has the characteristic large head and prominent forehead. The nose is broad and the cheeks are puffy. If the eyes were open, corneal opacification could be seen. The tongue is enlarged and the lips are thick. The facial features are generally coarse. Examination of the abdomen would reveal hepatosplenomegaly. This child had stiff joints and a gibbus, or hunchback, deformity of the thoracic spine.

The *Morquio syndrome* is also inherited as an autosomal recessive trait. The patient pictured here is an adult. (The scale is in centimeters.) She demonstrates the striking dwarfism (patients with the Morquio syndrome are rarely more than 4 feet tall) and lumbar lordosis seen in this syndrome. Her thoracic cage has a large AP diameter.

The upper extremity is proportionally more shortened than the lower extremity. The knees are held in the genu valgum position (knock-knees). Unlike patients with the Hurler syndrome, whose joints are stiff, the Morquio patients have increased range of motion. This patient was quite normal mentally. Hearing disorders develop in some patients as they grow older.

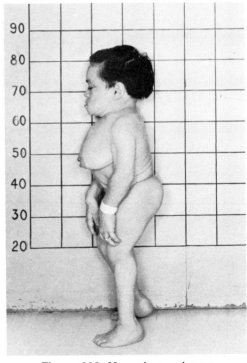

Figure 298. Morquio syndrome

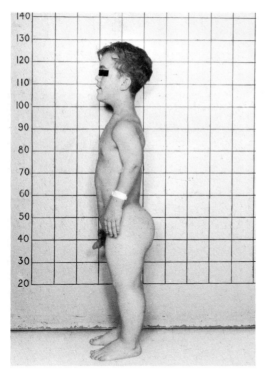

Figure 299. Achondroplasia

Achondroplasia is the most common type of dwarfism. It is inherited as an autosomal dominant trait, but seven out of eight cases occur as new mutations. Clinically these patients have a large head with frontal bossing. The nasal bridge is shallow. The chest and abdomen may be normal, but sometimes the abdomen appears protuberant. The gluteal region is prominent because of exaggerated lumbar lordosis; the upper and lower extremities are equally shortened, and the fingers are stubby. The mental capability usually is normal, dull-normal, or slightly more retarded.

Pycnodysostosis, an uncommon cause of dwarfism, is inherited as an autosomal recessive trait. This young lady still had open anterior and posterior fontanelles. This illustration shows the characteristic receding chin, about which more will be said later. The girl was just under 5 feet tall. She had short fingers with dished out, or spoon-shaped, nails. Her problem clinically was that minimal trauma resulted in fractures. She was mentally normal.

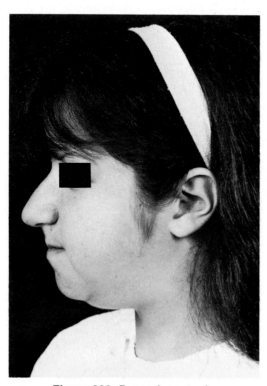

Figure 300. Pycnodysostosis

THE HURLER SYNDROME

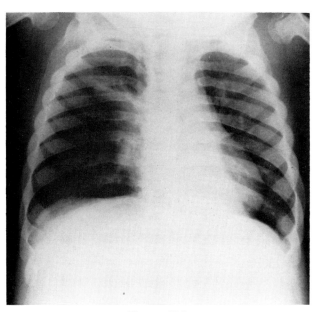

Figure 301.

Of the six mucopolysaccharidoses, the Hurler syndrome is the most widely known and occurs frequently. This child was 3 years old when these radiographs were made. At birth, the child seemed normal. The mental deterioration and grotesque facial features were present by the end of the first year.

The chest radiograph shows ribs that are wider than the interspaces. There is a characteristic narrowing near the vertebral column (paddle-shaped ribs). The heart may become enlarged when mucopolysaccharide deposition occurs in the myocardium and the valves. When the cardiac enlargement compresses the left lower lobe bronchus, atelectasis results, as seen here. (There is also a plaque of atelectasis in the right upper lobe.) One of the frequent problems seen in the Hurler syndrome is recurrent pneumonia.

The hand radiograph demonstrates delayed ossification of the carpal bones, proximal pointing of the second through fifth metacarpals, and broadening of the metacarpals and phalanges. The distal ends of the radius and ulna are angulated obliquely, so that they slant toward each other.

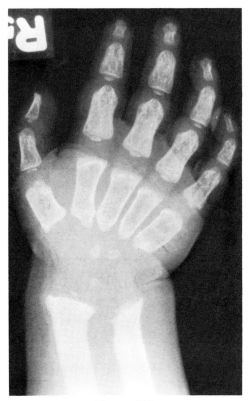

Figure 302.

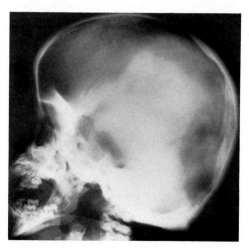

Figure 303.

The skull radiograph (Fig. 303) demonstrates the characteristic thickening of the skull base, large cranial vault, frontal bossing, fusion of the sutures, and a "J-shaped" or "omega" sella turcica. (The J-shaped sella is seen in a number of conditions, including in the normal infant. Actually, it refers to depression of the sulcus chiasmatis and planum sphenoidale, leading to a fancied resemblance to the letter J. It was shown by Neuhauser that arachnoid cysts are responsible for the formation of the J-shaped sella in the Hurler syndrome.) Notice that the mandible is short and that the third molars are seated on the ramus.

The vertebral bodies (Fig. 304) have a concave posterior scalloping, with pedicles that are longer than normal. The first lumbar vertebra is hypoplastic and is situated posterior to the other vertebrae, thereby creating a gibbus deformity (hunchback). There is a tongue or beak of the inferior aspect of the upper lumbar vertebrae that protrudes anteriorly. This is a characteristic finding.

The radiograph of the pelvis (Fig. 305) reveals flared iliac wings and constriction of the body of the iliac bone with an almost imperceptible dimple (or "spicule") at the lateral margin of the acetabulum. This leads to subluxation of the hips. There is also bilateral coxa valga and delayed ossification of the capital femoral epiphyses.

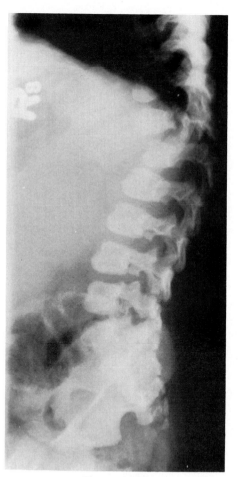

Figure 304.

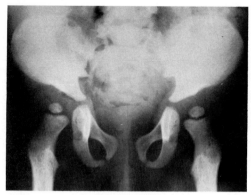

Figure 305.

THE MORQUIO SYNDROME

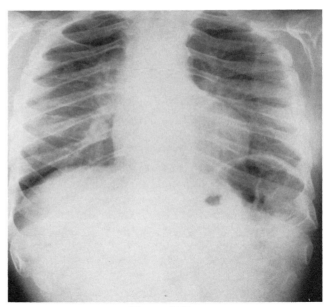

Figure 306.

Patients with the Morquio syndrome differ from those with the Hurler syndrome in several important ways. The Morquio patients are usually normal mentally, whereas the Hurler patients are profoundly and increasingly retarded. The Morquio patients excrete keratan sulfate in the urine; the Hurler patients excrete dermatan sulfate and heparan sulfate. Both types of patients are strikingly dwarfed. The Hurler patients have marked corneal opacification, but this is milder in the Morquio patients. The Hurler patients do not survive nearly as long as the Morquio patients. In fact, one of the original patients described by Morquio was 54 years old in 1971! The patient seen here was 16 years old when these radiographs were made.

The chest (Figs. 306 and 307) has a marked pectus carinatum deformity and an increased AP diameter. The ribs are wide, especially anteriorly, and do not project over the sternum (on the lateral view).

The wrists are swollen, and the hands are malformed (Fig. 308). Delayed ossification is seen. Other features of the hand radiograph include small carpal bones and proximal pointing of the second through fifth metacarpals. Because the ulna is shortened, there is ulnar deviation of the hands. Compare these radiographs with those of the other dystrophies.

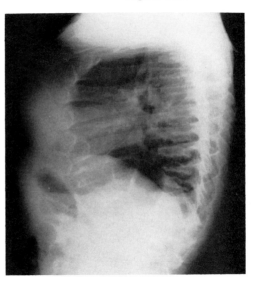

Figure 307.

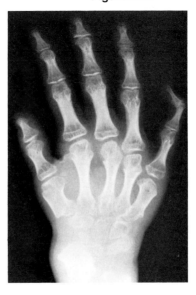

Figure 308.

All of the vertebrae are flattened (platyspondyly). The lateral view of the cervical spine (Fig. 309) shows that the odontoid process is absent. The atlas is held close to the occiput, and upon flexion the atlas slips anteriorly over the axis. It is not surprising that one of the common causes of death is atlantoaxial dislocation, resulting in spinal cord compression.

In the lower dorsal and upper lumbar spine (Fig. 310) there is an anterior beak in the *middle* of the vertebral body. (In the Hurler syndrome the anterior beak is seen in the inferior or *hind* part of the vertebral body. M = middle = Morquio. H = hind = Hurler.)

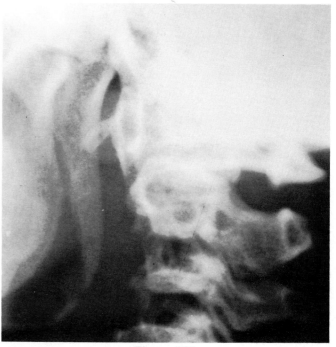

Figure 309.

The pelvis (Fig. 311) shows marked narrowing of the iliac body. The acetabula are not well formed, and the hips are dislocated. The capital femoral epiphyses undergo changes that resemble aseptic necrosis and then eventually disappear. The femoral necks show a valgus deformity and become widened and fragmented.

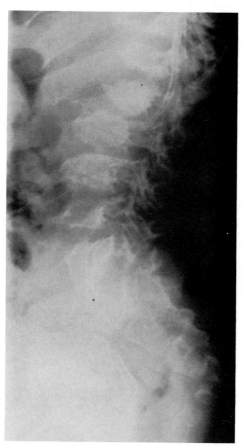

Figure 310.

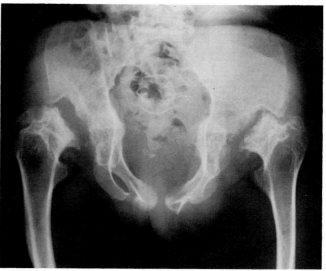

Figure 311.

ACHONDROPLASIA

This patient was 7 months old at the time that these radiographs were made. The view of the lumbar spine (Fig. 312) is almost diagnostic of achondroplasia because the distance between the pedicles decreases between the first and fifth lumbar vertebrae. Normally the interpediculate distance increases in this region. A lateral view of the lumbar spine would show shortened pedicles. It is not surprising that nerve root compression is seen frequently in patients with achondroplasia because of the diminished volume of the spinal canal.

The pelvis (Fig. 313) has squared iliac wings with a very narrow greater sciatic notch. The acetabular roofs are not quite horizontal.

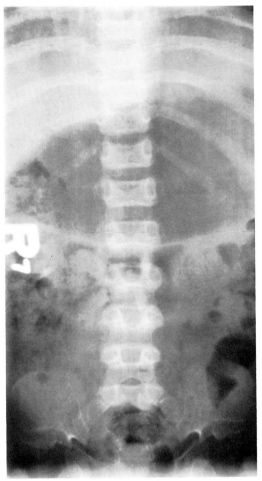

Figure 312.

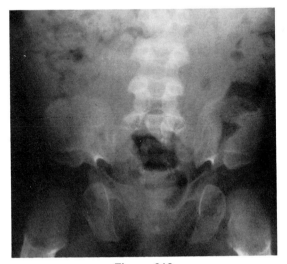

Figure 313.

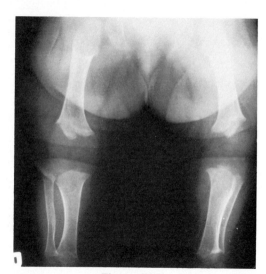

Figure 314.

The long bones of the extremities (Fig. 314) are shortened, and their metaphyses flare. The epiphyses of the distal femora appear to be sunken into the metaphyses. This change will develop in the proximal tibial epiphyses as well. In older children, the fibula is longer than the tibia; this may result in inversion of the feet.

The base of the skull is foreshortened, whereas the membrane-formed vault is relatively large. The frontal region is characteristically prominent. The foramen magnum is small and is usually hidden in the normally positioned Towne's projection (Fig. 316). Some of the patients with achondroplasia develop mild hydrocephalus, probably of the communicating type. The hydrocephalus has been ascribed to the small foramen magnum, but the actual mechanism is probably much more complex.

The hands have a stubby, shortened appearance. If the middle and ring fingers are separated, the term "trident hand" is used.

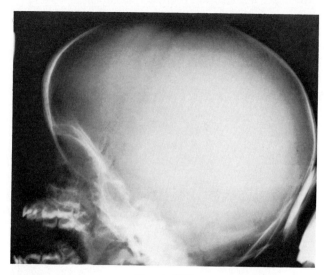

Figure 315.

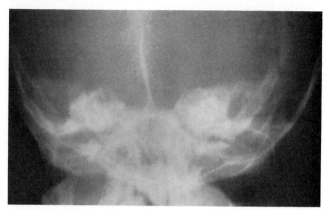

Figure 316.

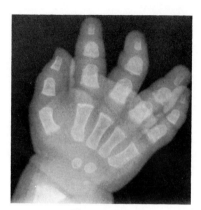

Figure 317.

PYCNODYSOSTOSIS

The last of the skeletal dysplasias to be discussed here is pycnodysostosis. This condition is characterized by short stature (rarely are the patients more than 5 feet tall), dense bones that fracture easily, skull and mandible anomalies, and hypoplasia or absence of the terminal phalanges.

The base of the skull (Figs. 318 and 319) appears thick. The sutures are widely separated, the fontanelles are large, and sometimes wormian bones are seen. The sinuses are frequently poorly developed. The angle of the mandible is straight (Fig. 319).

The long bones (Fig. 320) are dense, as seen in the distal radius and ulna. The hand radiograph also shows the striking hypoplasia of the distal phalanges and the lack of the ungual tufts. The fingernails are frequently spoon-shaped and clubbed.

Clinically, fractures are the biggest problem. Trauma that wouldn't be remembered in a normal child causes fractures in children with pycnodysostosis. Unlike in patients with osteopetrosis, anemia is not a problem.

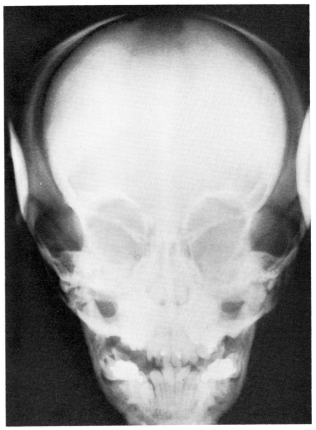

Figure 318.

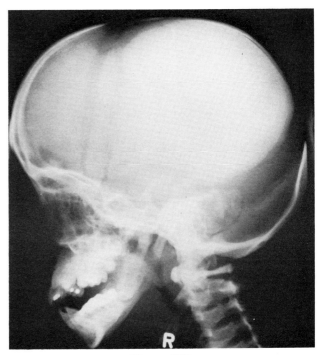

Figure 319.

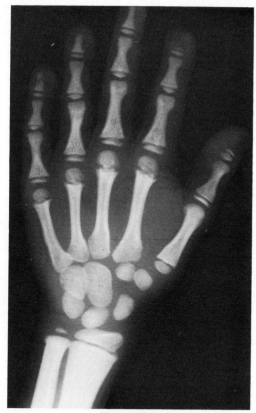

Figure 320.

This condition is interesting because it is now thought that the artist Henri de Toulouse-Lautrec suffered from pycnodysostosis. The evidence is reviewed in an article by Maroteaux and Lamy (J.A.M.A. 191:715–717, 1965). They point out that skeletal injuries prevented Toulouse-Lautrec from horseback riding, and his attentions were directed toward painting quite early. He suffered two known fractures from insignificant trauma. His fingers were very short and stubby, and his height was 4 feet 2 inches.

One of the important features of pycnodysostosis is the appearance of the head. The mandible is small; Maroteaux and Lamy speculate that Toulouse-Lautrec grew a beard to cover his receding chin. The skull is large, with open sutures and fontanelles. Most of the pictures of Toulouse-Lautrec show him wearing a hat (Fig. 321). It is thought that he wore a hat to protect the open fontanelles.

The parents of patients with pycnodysostosis frequently are related, since pycnodysostosis is inherited as an autosomal recessive trait. Toulouse-Lautrec's parents were first cousins. There are no known radiographs, and therefore no absolute proof, but on the basis of parental consanguinity, short stature, skull configuration, stubby fingers, and the history of fractures, it seems likely that Henri had pycnodysostosis.

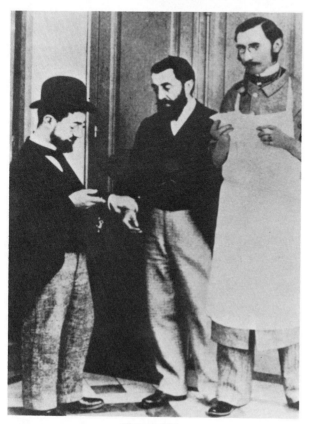

The short fellow is Henri.

(This figure courtesy of Knud W. Jensen, Director of The Louisiana Art Gallery, Humlebaek, Denmark.)

Figure 321.

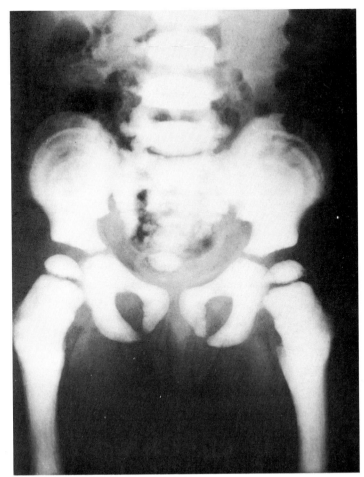

Figure 322. Peter D.

Peter **Densebone** has anemia and cranial nerve palsies.

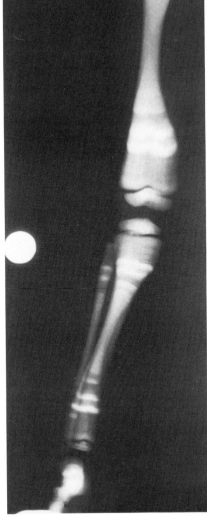

Figure 323. Peter D.

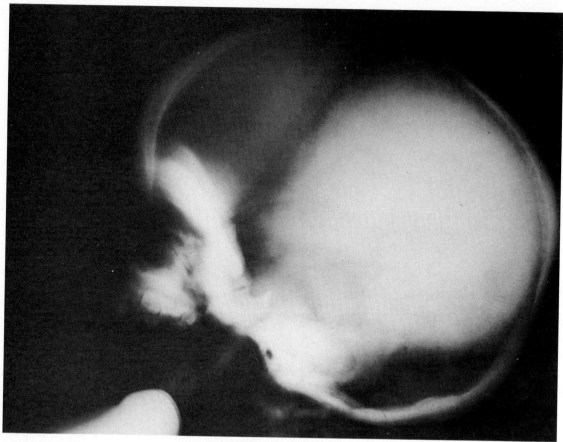

Figure 324. Peter D.

ANSWER

This selection of radiographs from a skeletal survey shows *extremely* radiopaque bones. Note the very constricted marrow space of the long tubular bones, which is responsible for *Peter's* anemia. Additionally, you should observe a "bone within bone" appearance, especially affecting the iliac wings and extremities. The skull base is very thickened, and narrowing of the basal foramina results in cranial nerve palsies.

This child has osteopetrosis, also known as "marble bones" or Albers-Schönberg disease. This disease, which is of unknown etiology, may be inherited in either a dominant or recessive form. In either case, osteopetrosis may be either mild in its manifestations and late in its presentation or relatively malignant in its manifestations (resulting mainly from severe anemia) and early in its presentation. The radiographic findings in osteopetrosis are very helpful in establishing the correct diagnosis.

Quiz

FINAL EXERCISE, REVIEW, AND ACROSTIC

Find among the following 15 illustrations the one that best tallies with each of the items below on this page, then enter the *letter designation of the figure* in the blank following the *corresponding historical item below*. When you have successfully completed the acrostic, you will have a comment we hope you'll make as you close the book.

ATTENTION: Figures may be used once, several times, or not at all.

1. Child with a complication of sickle cell disease .... _____

2. Child who presented with a history of bloody diarrhea without pain for six weeks .... _____

3. Baby with roentgen evidence of high small bowel obstruction ..... _____

4. Baby with roentgen evidence of low small bowel obstruction....... _____

5. Child with colicky right flank pain and hematuria for 24 hours.... _____

6. Child with episodes of diarrhea, fever, right lower quadrant pain, and tenderness... _____

7. Child with cough and roentgen evidence for a posterior mediastinal mass .... _____

8. Child with a right lower quadrant tender mass...................... _____

9. Child with plate-like atelectasis in the usual position of the minor fissure, secondary to the child's major problem...................... _____

10. Child with cough and roentgen evidence of croup .... _____

11. Child with unilateral ureteral obstruction and hydronephrosis... _____

12. Child with projectile vomiting... _____

13. Child with midline abdominal mass but no symptoms............... _____

14. Child with cough and roentgen evidence of left lower lobe collapse... _____

15. Child whose chest film shows rib erosion .... _____

16. Child with cough for six months and evidence of an endobronchial foreign body .... _____

17. Child whose intravenous urogram shows rotation of both kidneys .... _____

18. Newborn with choking and coughing upon first feeding............. _____

19. Child with cough and steatorrhea .... _____

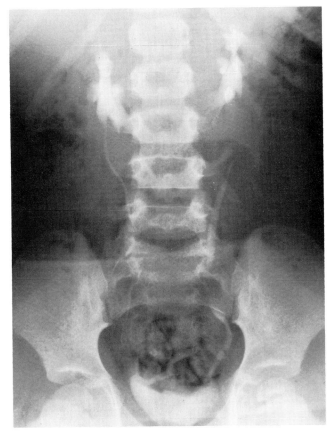

Figure L.

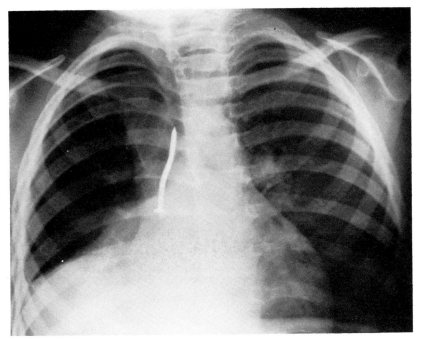

Figure P.

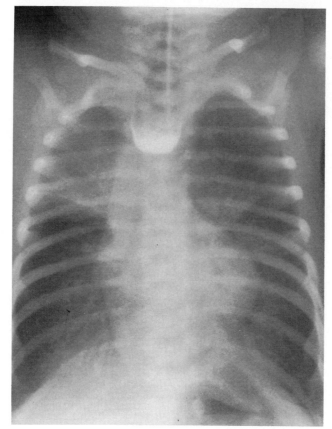

Figure A.

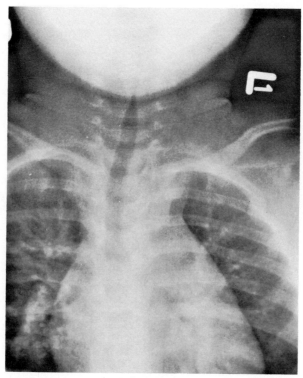

Figure C.

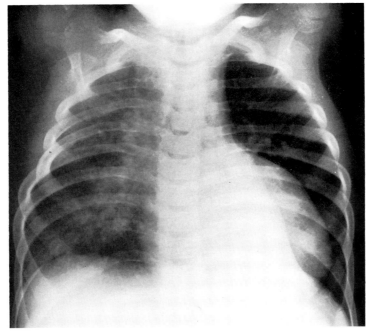

Figure D.

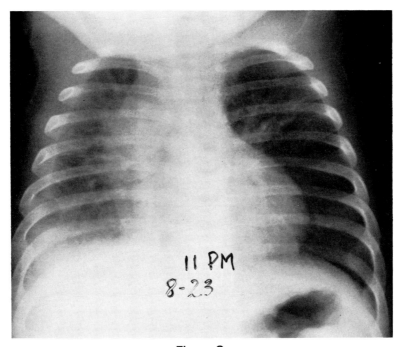

Figure G.

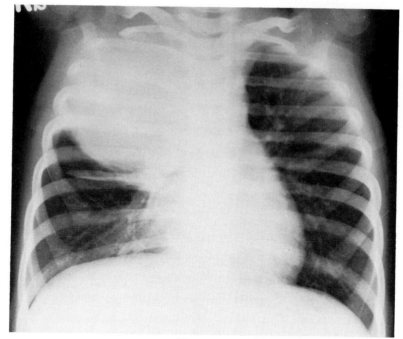

Figure S.

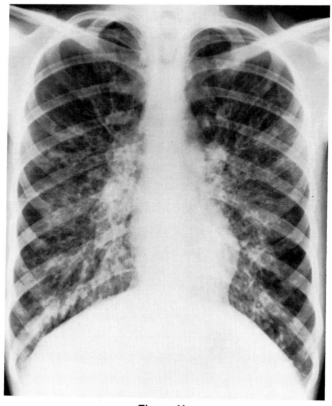

Figure Y₁.

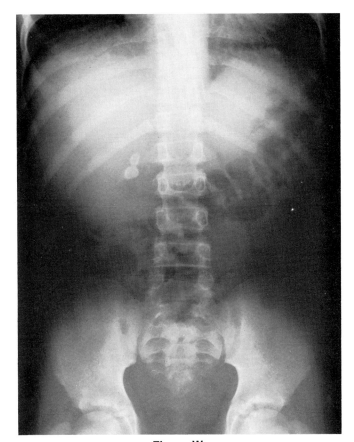

Figure W.

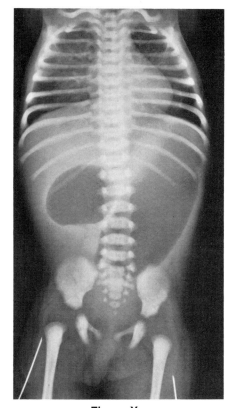

Figure Y₂.

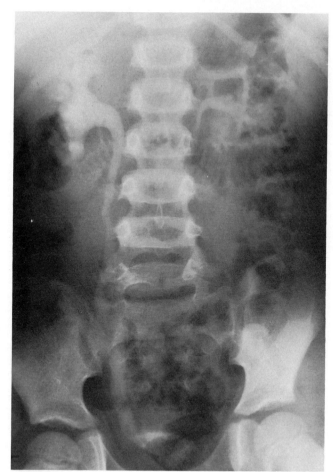

Figure H₁.

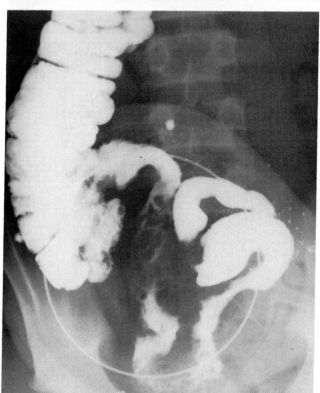

Figure I₁.

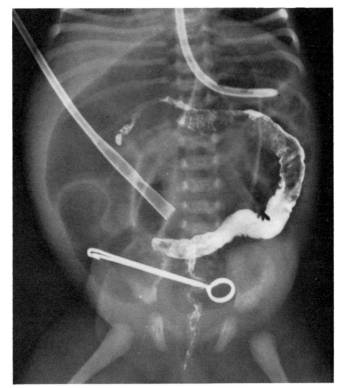

Figure T.

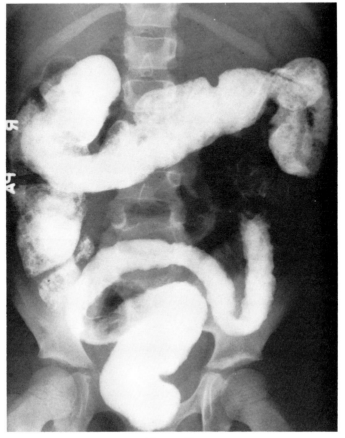

Figure H₂.

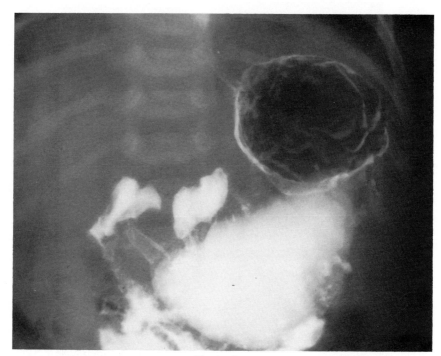

Figure I₂.

Answers to Quiz

ANSWERS

1. Gallstones in sickle cell disease.. W

2. Ulcerative colitis.. H_2

3. Double bubble in duodenal obstruction .... Y_2

4. Unused colon, dilated small bowel... T

5. Ureteral calculus at ureterovesical junction...................................... H_1

6. Regional enteritis... I_1

7. Ganglioneuroma .... S

8. (Same as 6) .... I_1

9. (Same as 7) compression atelectasis.. S

10. Croup... C

11. (Same as 5) .... H_1

12. Hypertrophic pyloric stenosis... I_2

13. Fused (horseshoe) kidney L

14. Left lower lobe collapse .... D

15. (Same as 7) .... S

16. Nail in the bronchus intermedius.. P

17. (Same as 13).. L

18. Esophageal atresia with atelectasis of upper lobes .... A

19. Cystic fibrosis.. Y_1

(G was not used but shows a pleural effusion in a baby with staphylococcal pneumonia.)

INDEX

NOTE: This is not really a formal index at all! Rather, it is simply meant to help you find something you want to see over again. Page numbers in **boldface** refer to page on which illustration may be found; those in lightface refer to discussion in the text.